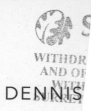

DENNIS

The Locked Ward

Memoirs of a Psychiatric Orderly

VINTAGE BOOKS
London

Published by Vintage 2013

2 4 6 8 10 9 7 5 3 1

First published in Great Britain in 2012 by
Jonathan Cape

Vintage
Random House, 20 Vauxhall Bridge Road,
London SW1V 2SA

www.vintage-books.co.uk

Addresses for companies within The Random House Group Limited
can be found at: www.randomhouse.co.uk/offices.htm

The Random House Group Limited Reg. No. 954009

A CIP catalogue record for this book
is available from the British Library

ISBN 9780099554356

The Random House Group Limited supports The Forest Stewardship
Council (FSC®), the leading international forest certification
organisation. Our books carrying the FSC label are printed on FSC®
certified paper. FSC is the only forest certification scheme endorsed
by the leading environmental organisations, including Greenpeace.
Our paper procurement policy can be found at:
www.randomhouse.co.uk/environment

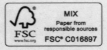

Printed and bound by CPI Group (UK) Ltd, Croydon, CR0 4YY

I am never better than when I am mad.
Then methinks I am a brave fellow;
then I do wonders. But reason abuseth me,
and there's the torment; there's the hell.

Thomas Kyd, *The Spanish Tragedy*

Though they go mad, they shall be sane;
Though they sink through the sea, they shall rise again.

Dylan Thomas, 'And Death Shall Have No Dominion'

Preface

Some years ago I was working in a Geriatrics ward in a Scottish hospital when I was headhunted by the Charge Nurse of the Intensive Psychiatric Care Unit, a man who had known me for some time. A previous staff member had proved unsatisfactory, a replacement was necessary and the Charge Nurse had requested that I be transferred to him.

'I don't know if I'm the man you want,' I told him. 'I can't fight.'

'I don't need fighters,' he replied. 'I need people who can listen.'

That conversation revealed much about my ignorance and suspicion, not to mention fear, of the ward. I was to learn very quickly that, while some degree of restraint is occasionally required in such a unit, the ability to share a fellow human being's burden is far more important. But it made me think. If I was so naive and misinformed – I who worked in psychiatry – how much more so would the general public be? Which is why, now that I have left the service, I've written this memoir.

Let me make it clear that the patients I helped nurse are not the people the reader will meet in these pages. Names, ages, nationalities, even the genders, of patients and staff have been changed to ensure complete confidentiality. The patients in the book are all fictions; fictions that allow me to discuss from direct experience mental illnesses, how they affect people and how they are treated. I spent too long trying to gain people's trust and help them rebuild their identities to betray all of that work now. Similarly, my colleagues on the ward make no appearance in these pages. They do difficult and stressful work in a dedicated fashion for little remuneration, and the last thing they need is to find themselves in a book. I have used fictional names and made no reference to the comings and goings of staff over the period. So, in short, the people are fictions, the illnesses and symptoms are typical, while the incidents and emotions are real.

I worked in the Locked Ward for seven and a half years. The job I feared turned out to be life-enhancing, heart-warming, heart-breaking, sometimes grim, occasionally terrifying and often funny. Funny? Yes, extremely so at times. But my purpose in writing is not to poke fun at anyone, nor to encourage any view of psychiatric illness as a nineteenth-century freak show. Some of these people were the smartest I ever came across.

I have written the memoir for several reasons. First, it was by far the most interesting job I ever had, and I believe others will find it interesting. Second, without being a psychiatric textbook, I hope it will inform people about the nature of serious mental illness and how it is treated. I hope it will correct misconceptions, and show that people with serious mental illness can say or do funny things, sad things or bad things; be brave, resolute, irritating, selfish, generous, kind, cruel or petty just like everybody else. Mainly, though, I want it to *celebrate* a group of people who are misunderstood, mistrusted or viewed with apprehension – the patients.

Because patients are not just people *like* you and me; they *are* you and me – you and me and the guy next door, and the girl you went out with, and your brother and sister, and mother and father, and son and daughter – just people who happen, sometimes once in their lives, sometimes on a chronic basis, to contract a psychiatric illness. It's been estimated that a third of us will meet the criteria for a major psychiatric illness at some point in our lives. All of us know stress, anxiety and hopelessness. The fears and concerns, hopes and despairs experienced by patients are experienced by the rest of us. Sometimes it's just a question of degree. Salvador Dali said, 'The only difference between me and a madman is that I am not mad.' I kind of know what he meant.

I hope the book is full of humanity as well as humour. But the two are always inseparable.

1

Why should not old men be mad?
W.B. Yeats

I called them 'loonies' as a child. But then everyone did.

Loonies were the strange and fearful people who hung about the bus stop outside the old asylum on the city bus route. They had faces like demons from medieval paintings. They gibbered and grimaced, made mouths and chattered as if they were suffering the agonies of the damned. What I didn't know then was that they probably were. I was a child: I didn't know any better. But they terrified me with their long, sickly faces and their unpredictable behaviour. They were part of the secret fauna of my nightmares.

Loonies. Lunatics. Men with the moon in their heads. I had first heard the word from a classmate in the 1950s. I think it may have been during my very brief flirtation with the Cubs, for the conversation took place in the old school playground on a summer's evening, long after school hours. An old man was hobbling painfully along the pavement on the sunlit side of the road opposite the yard. He was burly, with a heavy winter coat on, and he was carrying a shopping bag. The shops had all been shut for hours. His face was bright red. But what drew my attention to him was the leather helmet he wore: a close-fitting soft leather thing, slightly peaked, with a strap buckled tight under his chin. The sort of thing boys wore. It didn't look right on an old man. It looked incongruous. I didn't know the word then, although I had a good vocabulary and could spell 'syzygy', but I knew the feeling. Something was definitely somewhere else.

'Hey,' I shouted. 'Look at the old boy with the helmet.'

'Here,' hissed a boy called Gemmell. 'Shh! Dinnae let him hear ye! That's auld Brennan. He's a loony.'

'A loony?'

'He's mad! He lives in an auld ruined hoose, an' he eats rats, an' he's always tryin' tae wangle kids intae his hoose. If ye kick yer ba' intae his gairden, ye jist leave it.'

I imploded with dread. It was *The Old Dark House* and every other terrifying Gothic horror story come to life and taking place in this 1950s backwater. I couldn't sleep for nights.

In the following years occasional whispers reached my ears: fleeting confidences, hints that loonies were not the isolated phenomenon I could have wished. I overheard snatches of conversation from parents and adult neighbours that chilled me. I heard about the 'mental wifie' whose man had left her and who sat in the living room at night, once the kids had gone to bed, singing hymns to the Virgin Mary while dressed in her Sunday best. I heard of the spinster who had nursed her elderly mother and then, when she died, had lost her wits and visited the grave every Sunday with a picnic lunch to share with her. She would sit by the grave and conduct a conversation with the air, as if her mother were still there. And the lawyer's son who went raving mad and had to be taken away to the asylum in a yellow van.

It was always a yellow van in the legends of my childhood. I never saw one. Anywhere. At any time. All the time I was growing up. But, everybody knew, loonies were trapped by men in white coats and carted off to the asylum in a yellow van.

Some years later, as a student, I took a vacation job in the asylum. I thought it would be cool and hip, an absurdist dream. It wasn't. Twerp that I was, I thought that what Samuel Beckett's writing and mental illness had in common was that they were alternative slants on reality. I thought it would be cool to work as a nurse in a psychiatric ward. Nowadays I know that while it might be true of Beckett's art, it is the grossest insult to people with mental illness to consider them as distorting views of a normal reality – human fairground mirrors.

It was hard graft. And it was a revelation. Even as a smart-arsed and (I thought) sophisticated twenty-year-old, my heart was pulled in twenty different directions. Those 'loonies' were still there, lying stiff and still as gargoyles on the beds or slithering around the walls, lurking in corners, breathing shadows. But they weren't demons now. They were the flotsam and jetsam of two generations previous, discarded by a society which had no use for them, abandoned by families who were ashamed of them. Reading through the bulky files that had accumulated on each of them over decades, I unearthed tale after tale of human tragedy: daughters locked away for having children out of wedlock; sons immured for compulsive gambling or alcoholism; children put into asylums for some physical condition that discredited them in the eyes of their parents; lives grown fetid and stale, minds rotted day by day over the slow lapse of the years.

These people had indeed suffered the agonies of the damned. They were grey and stone-faced because they were hopelessly institutionalised, knowing no home but the drab confines of the ward, and utterly reliant on the staff. And staff are just like everybody else, everywhere else: some are kind and compassionate, some detached and cold, some cruel and domineering. Some staff could be all of them in one day, depending on the mood they were in. But the patients depended on them completely. The patients had no life worth the name; they were husks. All the sap, all the goodness, all the hope in their lives had long ago dried out. It changed my attitude profoundly.

Far from being the National Health Service equivalent of *Waiting for Godot*, it was back-breaking work for thirteen hours a day. I started at 7.30 a.m. and finished at 8.30 p.m. with a one-hour lunch break in the middle. The wards were full of demented old men who needed to be roused in the morning; dressed, washed and shaved before breakfast; fed breakfast and then accompanied to the Dayroom; entertained and/ or medicated till lunchtime; fed lunch and cleaned up afterwards; returned to the Dayroom for their afternoon tedium; fed dinner and then undressed and pyjama-ed before being returned to bed. It was non-stop and exhausting.

I lived in a flat in the city. Starting work at 7.30 in the morning meant I had to get up at six, have a coffee and a fag, then catch a corporation bus to the terminus, where I caught a service bus out to the asylum. The same thing happened in reverse at night. I often got back to the flat after ten o'clock, when I had a coffee and a fag then put myself straight to bed. But it was a job I did find satisfying, the minute I dropped the arty-farty fantasies. I felt I was actually contributing something to society for once. And there were some fine characters among the patients, some of whom I grew very fond of.

There was Abie. Abie's real name was Ebenezer, which was enough to endear him to me on its own. He had been a soldier, a pipe major who had led his band at the Edinburgh Tattoo at some dim and distant time. Now he was hardly military in bearing. He had a floppy crest of silver-white hair and a curious bird-like hopping gait. And he was extremely annoyed by my coiffure. Shoulder-length hair, I knew, would be a positive drawback on the ward so at my interview I had offered to tie it back in a ponytail – still something of a sissy novelty in those days. That was jessie enough but the senior nursing officer, a vinegar-titted old bag, insisted not only that it be tied back, the ponytail should also be kirby-gripped. With the result that I wafted about the ward with a hairstyle not unlike a chignon or a French twist. It is not hard to imagine how much this would appeal to an ex-pipe major. The first time he clapped eyes on me, Abie was hirpling back from the lavatory with a bale of toilet tissue stuffed down his jacket. He saw me, stopped dead on one leg like a startled stork, clapped one palm several times very rapidly against his brow and hissed 'Hair like a wumman!' I elicited this reaction every time he saw me, the whole time I was there.

Magnus from Paisley was skeletally thin, appeared like a phantom from behind curtains or by the side of cupboards, and had a gravelly voice several octaves lower than that of an Aberdeen Angus. In his sepulchral tones he would inform you as you passed by, 'Ah'm the king ae Egypt.' Quite what he based that on, I never knew. I never saw him wear a striped towel on his head or sport a tie-on beard. He never walked like an Egyptian, and his surname was not Ptolemy. But, several times a week, I'd pass Magnus having a quiet lurk in a corner and he'd rumble, 'Ah'm the king ae Egypt.' Actually, I always thought Magnus was a lot less daft than he cracked on to be. Often I caught him earwigging outside the office door or eavesdropping on other staff conversations.

He'd move on with a shifty grin when caught, but he never acted as demented as the other old men. Maybe he felt he had to sound unhinged every so often, to keep his place. I got the distinct impression that he was amusing himself at our expense.

Once, he gave himself a new role, perhaps tired of being typecast. One morning when I was in the Bathroom, running a bath for another patient, Magnus materialised at my elbow in his pyjamas, and informed me, 'Ah'm Dracula.' I said to him, 'Time you were back in your coffin, then; it's daylight.' He gave a quick snicker and was gone.

Surprisingly perhaps for one so thin, he enjoyed his meals. There was nothing of him, in terms of body weight – if he'd fallen from the heavens, he wouldn't have sprung a mouse trap. But he could certainly pack it away at mealtimes. He was especially devoted to custard, and would stand up from the table, scraping his spoon around his emptied dish. 'Ony mair Cremola?' he would grate.

There was a man called John Bunyan. When I told him, perhaps a little condescendingly, one day that there had been a very famous writer named John Bunyan, he looked at me tolerantly and said, 'Aye. *Pilgrim's Progress*,' as if he'd heard that all his life. Maybe he had. He was an amazing cadger of cigarettes and, on the few occasions that he couldn't manage to mooch one, would simply roll up ten or twenty leaves of toilet paper and smoke that. You always knew when John had been smoking paper. His eyebrows would be smouldering and he looked like he was auditioning for a part in *Showboat*.

John Sweeney, from Edinburgh, was a little owl of a man with great round eyes in a round, bald head on top of a round ball of a body. He had been an Edinburgh bus driver 'oan the number ferteen fae Wavelston Dykes', as he informed me. This little snippet of his conversation highlights perfectly both his speech impediments. (He meant the number thirteen from Ravelston Dykes.) Throaty of voice too, he was an Auld Reekie Elmer Fudd. He was a genial little man and liked to reminisce about his days in the army. He had served in Egypt, which was boring except when they got to visit the casbah and such places to see the fleshpots, which he always described as 'nakit wimmin dancin' re cha-cha'. Occasionally, friction arose between John and Magnus over the subject of Egypt, usually when Magnus asserted, 'Ah'm the King ae Egypt,' to which John would retort, 'Ur ye fuck.'

'Whit would you ken aboot it?' Magnus would say.

'Ah ken aw wight. Don't you wowwy aboot that. Ah wis vere. Ah kin wear re 1914–15 fuckin' wibbon.'

Then there was Wull. Wull broke my heart. He was a tall man, stooped, with a vaguely professorial look about him, greyish-white hair receding slightly from the temples and swept back from his forehead. He was as melancholy as autumn and kept himself apart from the other patients. Every day he looked for his daughter to visit, and every day he was disappointed.

'Nurse, d'ye think mah lassie'll come the day?' he asked me twenty times a day. And twenty times a day, with a lump in my throat, I said I hoped so. And I certainly did. But it never happened.

Knowing, he would nod and stroll away.

The staff were as motley a crew as the patients. A dozen deckhands dressed as Harlequin couldn't have been motlier. There was a guy called Wilson, whose nose and top lip twitched as if they were constantly being caught on a fishing hook. He couldn't talk without one side of his face rippling. It was certainly a fair collection of facial tics. I don't know if it was a nervous reaction, but it was impossible to tell if he was as happy as a pig in shit or profoundly miserable. He had the same grimace for every emotion. There was a laid-back American student. His full name was something like Randolph K. Albuquerque, but he liked being called Randy. He walked around with his long hair tied back in a normal ponytail. How come *he* didn't have to wear his hair in a bun? I got stonkingly miffed at that. And there was a pod of fat married women with a singular style of utterance.

'Ah hud therty pairs a rubber knickers in that fuckin' cubburd and thiv aw WALKED!'

'Ah dinny mind shite. Naw, shite ah kin take. Shite and pish, that's nae bother. Jist dinny ask me tae clean up boke.'

I called them the Hippos. Randy called them the Three Fat Ladies. They were extremely capable and experienced nurses, with mountains of patience and affection for the patients in their care, but they looked down their noses at Randy and me. Students. Time-wasters. Just fannying around the ward for a few bob till next term started. That was what they thought of us. I could tell. At break time they'd sit on one side of the table like 888, smoke, swear and take the piss out of us, as we sat facing them.

'Student, are ye, son?' asked Hippo 3 my first morning.

'Yeah,' I answered.

'Aye. Ye'll be like the rest a them. Smokin' they drugs an' ridin' aw day.'

'Disnae look like he's got a ride in him,' ventured Hippo 1.

'Ach, there'll be wan ride in him,' opined Hippo 2, 'an' it'll be haudin' him thegither!'

They collapsed into wheezes of smoky laughter. Bless them.

There was also a teuchter – a Highlander – who was studying for a BEd – 'It's the deghree off the fewture' (No, it wasn't) – a handsome brown-skinned guy from Mauritius called Sid and a bald middle-aged man from Glasgow called Tam. Tam was as gay as a thrush. Sid's real name may have been something Islamic like Siddiqi, or something even more esoteric like Siddartha Gautama. But he got 'Sid'. What he also got was Tam. Tam spanieled around the place in Sid's wake. Everywhere that poor Sid went, Tam was sure to go. Where Sid worked, Tam worked too. When Sid took his lunch, Tam took lunch right alongside him. Tam got to talking about 'me an' Sssid' like they were an old couple.

'Me an' Sssid jisst cheynged the auld boay an 'oor ago, an' he's covert in ssshite again!

'Look, that's ssstrange that, eh, intit? Ye dinnae see minny folk wae Sssid's skin colour thit's goat freckles, daen't ye no? But there wan right there, look, oan his cheekbone.'

There was no doubt in my mind what interested Tam in Sid's freckle.

We worked New Year's Day. Tam told me that he had been up 'aw night' partying and carousing. When we asked him if he'd had any sleep, he replied like Danny La Rue, 'Ah'd half an 'oor in the big chair.'

Wilson came in, grimacing and twitching, and asked Tam how he'd got on. Had he been drunk? Had he slept?

'Ah'd half an 'oor in the big chair.'

Any time I passed Tam in conversation, for the rest of that day, even if it was in a corridor, emptying a laundry basket, or changing an old guy's clothes in the ward, he was telling somebody, 'Ah'd half an 'oor in the big chair.'

Maybe it was a code.

It was while I was working there that I saw my first dead body. More than just saw it. Seeing it would have been all right, after the first shock.

It belonged to a patient named Laird, a huge man who had recently been admitted to the ward. Apart from his dementia, he was obviously very physically sick too. His admission probably had much to do with giving his exhausted wife some respite. He lay in the bed closest to the duty room. His breathing was poor, accompanied by much wheezing and gasping. It was one Sunday night, about seven o'clock, while his wife was sitting with him, that he died – horribly, coughing up mouthfuls of blood. I was alerted to the fact that something was wrong by his wife's piercing shriek from behind the screens. Unbelievably, there were only two of us on at the time – myself and the charge nurse, Benny. It being Christmas time, and the ward having been quiet, Benny had let everyone else go home. Benny took it upon himself to console Mr Laird's wife and escort her from the scene, while I phoned the duty doctor to come and certify death.

The doctor arrived and made it official that Laird was dead. Then Benny and I were left with him. Benny looked at me.

'Ah know you're only a student,' he said, 'and you'd have every right tae refuse, but ah need somebody tae assist me in dressin' the body.'

I took off like the Road Runner but all I could do was sprint very fast on the spot. Benny had a grip of the tails of my white coat. He leaned over my shoulder and informed me that there was nobody else he could ask. Benny was a decent guy and I felt I owed it to him to hang around – maybe even owed it to Mr Laird. So I said yes.

The ward was quiet, most of the night lights dimmed. The patients were in bed. We slipped the brakes off Mr Laird's bed and wheeled it out. The corridor, equally faintly lit, stretched silently away into the dim distance. We wheeled the bed into a side room. Benny flicked on the side lights and told me to stay with the body while he went and fetched the materials he would require to perform the grisly task. Then he went. And there was I, left in a silent side room, off a ghostly corridor, in an almost deserted asylum, in the depths of a dark and moonless winter's night, with the first stiff I had ever clapped eyes on. Mr Laird was under a sheet in the traditional way, but I was awfully conscious that he was a dead person, and the thought was not comforting.

The plastic doors to the side room were of the swing variety. I strode to them, pulled them towards me and stuck my head out into the corridor, holding the doors close to my chest. Thus I had my head out in the light and my arse in the gloom towards the late Mr Laird. Occasionally, for Benny wasn't quick about his errand, my skin would creep horribly and I was forced to turn and take a sneaky peek at the bed behind me. Just to make sure that Mr Laird hadn't moved in some ghastly, afterlife version of Statues. If he had sat up under his sheet and moaned, I would either have dropped dead myself or just run through doors, walls and anything else in my way, leaving a perfect me-shaped hole in each of them, like a cartoon.

This was bad enough. But then Benny returned and things got a damn sight worse. In those days registered nurses like Benny had to do the things for the deceased that are now done by undertakers. I won't go too far into the subject; I know many people are squeamish – I'm certainly one of them, and the memory of the procedure is as distressing as the original experience. Orifices have to be plugged – need I say any more? Other things have to be done, and they are best left to the imagination.

But they weren't, that night. I had to be present and assist Benny when he needed assisting. My contribution consisted mainly of passing things when requested, and watching with saucer eyes. The whole operation depressed the Dundee damn out of me. Eventually, the job was done and we heard the night shift come clattering in.

My walk to the bus stop on the main road that night, as every night, took me through the thickly wooded grounds. The darkness gathered around. I thought of crows and rooky woods. The only lights were the wan and witch-like lights of the various wards on the hill. My footsteps rang in the frosty air. My eyes flicked all over the trees and shrubs, on the lookout for I know not what. I had the ears of an African elephant, as they strained for any sound of ghost or ghoul come to snatch me from the upper world.

On my last day in the ward I had occasion to go upstairs for some errand I've now forgotten – to fetch linen or something – and walked in on Randy shagging one of the Hippos in a cupboard. He had obviously indulged in some foreplay, for she had her skirt up, her knickers round one ankle and her top down to her waist. She was bent over, gripping a shelf, with her breasts swinging under her like bells, while Randy, trousers at his ankles, was saddled up doggy style and banging away like a riveter. Neither of them even knew I was there. I shut the door and left them to it. Maybe she didn't despise him after all.

I said goodbye to Wull with a lump in my throat. I said goodbye to John and to the king of Egypt. I even said goodbye to Abie, but he just cocked his head like a macaw and hissed, 'Hair like a wumman!' And that was it. I felt I had done something worthwhile for once in my life, but it was time to go back to university and English literature. I handed in my white coat. I unpinned my tresses and threw away my kirby grips. I wouldn't be needing them for a while.

2
_____

The satirical rogue says here that old men have grey beards, that their faces are wrinkled, their eyes purging thick amber and plum-tree gum, and that they have a plentiful lack of wit, together with most weak hams: All which, sir, though I most powerfully and potently believe, yet I hold it not honesty to have it thus set down, for you yourself, sir, should be old as I am if, like a crab, you could go backward.

William Shakespeare, *Hamlet*

And that was the reason why, thirty years after all of that, when I eventually prised myself free from a job I had grown to loathe, I went back to Psychiatry. I didn't need the kirby grips this time. I had nothing left to pin up.

As I had before, I worked as an orderly, or nursing assistant (NA), in a Psychogeriatrics ward. But the term 'psychogeriatrics' was no longer in vogue. The service was now known as Care of the Elderly. Not that it made any difference to the people who mattered. That was part of the mim-mouthed renaming of things that went on in many professions, as if the substitution of euphemisms for slightly distasteful aspects of the job, by that simple act, removed them. It didn't of course, but the process was considered worthwhile – the intention was good, so the end result must be – therefore it continued. So patients were now known as 'clients', as though they were consulting a lawyer or a town planner, and as though they had popped into a psychiatric ward entirely of their own volition. It didn't make the slightest difference to their illnesses or the treatment they received, but it probably gave some Jack or Jill in government an excuse to draw a salary.

I worked in the elderly ward, one of six people on the shift, and the only male. We nursed twenty old men with dementia. As I'd found out thirty years before, the work is intensely task-driven. Starting at 7.30 in the morning, each man had to be woken up, washed, shaved and dressed. Some of the old men did not want to be woken up. Or washed. Or shaved. Or dressed. The older I get, the more I sympathise with them. Some of them didn't understand what was going on. And some of them fought fiercely against it. I was blootered more than once when I was kneeling to tie a patient's laces or trying to pull a shirt over another one's head.

Old men with dementia can be twitchy or prone to sudden, jerky movements. That was a lot of fun when I was trying to shave them without slicing their noses off. This was the end of the twentieth century, but the idea of electric razors did not seem to have permeated as far as the hospital. I had to use those awful plastic disposable things. Because they were cheap. And they were cheap because they were bloody useless. Even split new from the packet, they tore lumps off the old guys' faces and gouged holes in their chins. It was as if someone had been whittling wood with the razors before they were packaged up, or using them to scrimshaw fancy patterns on whales' teeth. They might have been the ticket for creative work, but for shaving they were worthless. And I was a poor barber.

But it was an aspect of the job I got good at. I washed their faces and shaved them when they were still lying in bed. With strugglers or fighters, I developed the ability to duck and bob like Muhammad Ali, darting back in under the swipe for another nonchalant scrape. Some nurses liked to tuck the sheets tight around the arms of fighters for the few moments it took to shave them. But it couldn't stop them from rolling their heads around and they still ended up with a face covered with white squares of paper with red circles. Some patients looked like a Japanese gala day.

Each patient was bathed once a week, according to a rota. That was even harder work, because many of them panicked in a bath full of water. They didn't know what was happening; they weren't prepared for it, so they were frightened. They struggled and kicked and splashed and slid about the bath. There were two of us but it was still a slog.

What I hadn't realised – one of the many things I hadn't realised – was that, although their minds were fading away, many of these old men still retained quite startling upper-body strength. They had been miners and foundry men, farmers and railway workers. Some of them had the chests of bulls and arms like my thighs. When they blootered you, you stayed blootered.

Most of the patients were incontinent and wore pads or nappies which had to be changed in the morning and regularly during the course of the day. It wasn't the best aspect of the job, dealing with shit, but it was a supremely necessary one, and one that quickly became routine. Sometimes more than routine. After a few weeks I discovered an unsuspected talent in myself. I got so that when I walked into the ward not only could I tell by the smell that someone had shit, I could often tell who it was. Now that's what I call a nose. What a loss I must have been to wine-making. Or perfumery.

Once up and dressed, the patients had to be escorted or wheeled to the dining room for breakfast. Some needed to be fed, a job that required patience and compassion.

And the ability to dodge blows again. Not everybody felt like porridge every morning. Sometimes you wore it. Please sir, I want some less. Thereafter, some were taken to the lounge and sat in big geriatric chairs. This is the image many associate with care homes and wards like mine: old folk motionless in chairs, faded like old photographs in sunlight. It wasn't that we didn't care. We hadn't time. We still had the rest of the ward to wake, wash, shave and dress, then take to breakfast. It took all morning. Daytime TV burbled gently in the background but few, if any, of the patients paid it any attention. It was as remote from their diminished reality as anything else in the present.

And the present was all that existed.

Dementia robs the sufferer gradually of his or her memories. It may be a comparatively slow process – it usually is – but it is an inexorable one. And a pitiless one. It starts with recent memories. Short-term memory loss is usually the first sign: 'I can remember every day of my childhood but I can't remember what the hell I had for lunch today.' So the days get pared away from the memory, and then the months and the years. But from the wrong direction – not the one you would expect. It happens backwards. Finally, the memory is erased completely.

Each patient had a cork pinboard above the locker by the side of his bed, and loved ones were encouraged to pin up old photographs of him and his family as a way of personalising an impersonal situation, of giving him a slight wisp of home and familiarity in the place. Weddings, holidays, family outings, all in black and white like stills from ancient movies, but movies that nobody could remember, with actors and actresses vaguely familiar, though nobody could quite place them or what they were in before.

We often tried to engage the men in conversation about their wives, their families or what they used to do for a living. It was a regular part of the routine. I learned a great deal – often about myself as much as about them. How much we had in common, and how fragile were our certainties. Often they could remember nothing. Or, if they could, they had no way of telling me about it. It was grievous. These old men, most of them in their seventies or eighties, had lived full lives, worked all their days, been servicemen during the war, brought up children, had grandchildren and even great-grandchildren. And knew nothing about it. They lived in a constant present, with no discernible connection to the past. They were living Groundhog Day. Every day was everyday. Each day was their first day. And they would never escape, never get better. The only way out was death. The ward was an elephants' graveyard.

Some patients walked around the corridors all day. Ceaselessly. Looking for something they couldn't remember and wouldn't have been able to recognise if they'd found. From one end of the long ward to the other they walked, a never-ending coming and going of purposeless old men. Some would smile and give a greeting.

'Hi, Desmond,' I might say.

'Hello, son. Lovely day.'

And on he would go.

'Am I on the right road for the bus stop?' Johnny asked me several times a day. He wore a jacket and cap, had stout walking shoes on his feet and carried a package of his belongings under his arm.

'Aye, just keep on this road till you come to it,' I'd say.

Not cruel but kind. Joining him in his own reality. Any other reply would have been cruel. Telling him he was in a psychiatric ward and was losing everything to dementia? If he'd believed me – understood me – he wouldn't have thanked me for it. Holding a mirror up to dementia patients can be a merciless thing to do. I saw a colleague draw a patient, at his own request, one evening. The portrait was excellent, a very recognisable likeness, but the patient was horrified. He thought my colleague was playing a joke. In his own reality he was about forty years old. He didn't recognise the failing old man he saw in the drawing. So I entered Johnny's reality and directed him to the bus that would never come. Only one vehicle would ever come for him.

I'd meet him on the return journey and we'd go through the same dialogue. Eventually, I'd find him slumped in a geriatric chair, cap and jacket still on, sound asleep. And my throat would close a little. He reminded me of my grandfather. He used to walk a lot too.

I'd find Andy standing motionless in the corridor, angled strangely to the wall as if someone had set him down there and gone to look for the instruction book. Or like an enchanter had turned him to stone in a field while the hospital shot up around him, slick and quick as a screen saver: bricks zipping in lines to make walls, pipes whizzing along the ceiling, slates dealt onto the roof like cards. He just stood there, caught in a forest of thorns that had jumped out of his own head. If I turned him to face the corridor, he'd stand and look light years into the distance that way. When I came back, he was always gone.

Hughie scooted around the ward like someone had wound a key in his back. Then he stood, shuddering, ticking over, ready to go again, but going nowhere.

The medicine trolley came round as regularly as the ice-cream man: first thing in the morning, mid-morning, afternoon and evening. It was opened up and various happy pills were doled out – and a few biffs of the liquid cosh, where appropriate. Most of the patients glumly accepted the pill/pellet/tablet/syrup proffered and the slurp of watery orange juice to wash it down. It was just one of the inexplicable things that happened to them. But some were recalcitrant where meds were concerned. They'd clamp their mouths tight shut, grimace one way then the other away from the medicine, dip their heads down towards their chests, anything to avoid the intrusion. It was like trying to give a pill to a cat.

Laundry arrived and each garment had to be allotted to its rightful owner and hung up in his press. Everything had its owner's name sewn into it, like it belonged to a child viewed through the wrong end of the telescope of time. The fun part was the bag of assorted socks that accompanied every cage of laundry. Maybe a hundred socks, all to be sorted into pairs. What a lovely way to spend an evening. Can't think of anything else I'd rather do.

Lunchtime meant that all twenty patients were fed together, then returned to the lounge before staff got their own lunch. Afternoon brought cleaning tasks, sorting linen, taking part in group activities with the patients, and an official toileting round, in which, one by one, every man was taken to the toilet and had his pad changed, no matter how often this had been done for him throughout the day. This was another time to be wary. Most of the old men had no idea what was going on and would suddenly find themselves inexplicably in the toilet, their trousers being taken down and someone footering around their bits – usually a female, sometimes a young one. Affronted or enraged, they would hit out. Which was why I got the job of standing facing them and holding their wrists while a colleague did the necessary from behind: undoing trousers, whipping off pad, cleaning quickly but gently; replacing pad then trousers. Some of them still tried to lash out, and one had a habit of trying to kick my shins into puff candy. Fortunately, he found it difficult with his trousers around his ankles.

Visitors came mid-morning, mid-afternoon and in the evening.

Ah, like the man says, if you have tears, prepare to shed them now. Wives and daughters came, love and devotion firing them to it, bringing favourite sweeties and treats forgotten a lifetime ago. And hardly a one was recognised. Husbands and fathers looked at them as if they were the most impudent of strangers. But still they came and sat by the shell of the man they had once known. Though the body looked the same, the person they loved had long since left it. It was like visiting a grave.

Tommy's wife came twice a week, sometimes more. She would sit by his chair, holding his hand, while he stared straight ahead into the void. Sometimes a single fat tear rolled down her cheek. He never looked at her. Tommy never looked at anyone, staff or visitor. If you turned his face towards you, he was looking at the edge of the universe. He didn't look at his wife because he had no memory of her being his wife. They had got married late. For years they had tried to have a child, with no success. Then she had got pregnant. Their daughter was two when Tommy started to dement. Early-onset dementia is crueller and more remorseless. The sufferer deteriorates more rapidly. Tommy had no idea he had a daughter. He had been exultant when she was born, his wife told me. Said it made him complete.

On the other hand, there was Jim. Jim used to sit like a figure on a totem pole, unmoving and unmoved. His expression was utterly impassive. And then, some nights, his daughter would arrive and his face would flash into life with the kind of smile that creaked, gone rusty because it had hardly been used in years.

Sometimes visitors would complain – understandably – that their father was wearing someone else's trousers, or that another patient was wearing their husband's shirt. I would explain that some patients soiled themselves so regularly, or spilt food and drinks so often, that it was necessary to borrow clothing from another patient just to have them decently attired. The men had to have their dignity. You couldn't have someone's husband or father sitting improperly dressed. And every one of them was somebody's husband, father, grandfather or brother. Younger staff, sometimes new to the set-up, had to be reminded of that. They sometimes only saw a mental old bugger who talked gibberish and walked out of the Bathroom with his trousers on his head like a giant rabbit. But that was somebody's dad, someone who had once flown Spitfires during the war.

After dinner we got some of the patients undressed and back to bed before the night shift came in. The day came full circle. We left the ward at 8.30. Thirteen hours on. I had no difficulty sleeping at night. Again, I felt I was doing something worthwhile. I got to like all of the old men, and to be really fond of some of them.

But I loved Stefan.

He was a Pole. I read his notes. In his youth, like so many of his compatriots, he had fought against Nazism with the Allies and had stayed in the UK after 1945. Initially he had based himself in the Liverpool area but latterly moved to Scotland to work in the mines. He had no wife, so he advertised in a Polish newspaper for a woman to come over to Scotland to marry him. One did, a lady whose Polish name I don't remember. It was anglicised to Jean, in any case. They too had tried for a family for a long time with no success, so they adopted a son and called him Jan. They brought him up as their own, lavished love and tenderness on him, saw him to manhood. He died in his twenties of leukaemia.

It was obvious, from my first day on the ward, that Stefan had been a working man. Though old and ill, his upper torso and arms were still those of a man who had worked hard all his life. He was sweet-natured and patient, despite the many tribulations that his illness brought him. At one time he could speak English very well, but his dementia had erased much of his adult memory and he spoke mainly in his native Polish. So I learned a few phrases in that tongue. And what a reward to reap from that scant effort!

The smile that greeted my '*Dzien dobry*, Stefan' when I woke him each morning was seraphic. He started to call me Jan. Whether he genuinely thought I was the son he had lost many years before or was simply expressing gratitude and affection for my effort doesn't matter. It was inexpressibly moving. He would shuffle along beside me in the corridor, perfectly happy to be in my presence. When he sat in a tall geriatric chair facing the TV in the evening, I'd sit next to him as often as my duties allowed. Once, I offered him a Murraymint. He smiled and shook his head, then patted my hand and spoke affectionately in Polish.

'He jist loves you,' one of my female colleagues said.

Good. Maybe it eased his suffering a little to have me – or the ghost of his dead adopted son – by him.

I went to his funeral. At the service the priest, quoting one of Stefan's relatives, described him as 'a son of Poland, a hard-working man, a good man'. I can't think of a fitter, or finer, epitaph. There was no need for grandiose claims. How many of the great and the grand can claim as much?

Do widzenia, stary przyjaciel.

There is no cure for dementia. Modern drugs can slow down the rate of deterioration, but nothing cures it. The only treatment we can give sufferers is TLC. And plenty of it. Carers need to make sure sufferers are safe, warm, fed and kept clean. But the very process of caring at home for a loved one can be grinding. No one who hasn't nursed someone suffering from dementia can be fully aware of how draining and wearing it can be. Which is why many carers need regular respite and many organisations exist to provide it.

I worked in the ward for just under a year.

Then one day Charlie, the charge nurse of the IPCU, came to the ward and asked to talk to me. I knew Charlie through his brother, who was in the same pub quiz team as myself. He said that one of the male NAs in the IPCU had proved to be less than satisfactory, and had moved on. Charlie wanted to know if I would come over and join the staff at the Intensive Psychiatric Care Unit, Ward 25 in the new hospital. The difference between that and my current ward was the difference between night and cheese.

Most of the clients in the Locked Ward, as many outsiders called it, were young, and most, though not all, were male. All were sectioned under the Mental Health Act and there against their wills. Patients in the Locked Ward were acutely unwell. Seriously unwell. Some were there because they were a threat to themselves or other people. In other words, violent. I wasn't sure.

'I don't know if I'm the man you want,' I told Charlie. 'I can't fight.'

'I don't need fighters,' Charlie replied. 'I need people who can listen.'

'Listen?'

'The biggest part of the job is talking to patients. By which I mean listening to them. Helping them sort things out. Being a sympathetic ear. Acting on what you find. For their benefit.'

'Right.'

'I know you can do that.'

'Right.'

'Well, would you be interested? If nothing else, it would get you off the Shite Detail.'

'Yeah, I guess so. So long as I'm not going to be a punchbag.'

'You won't. We've got plenty of guys who can fight.'

That was intended as a joke.

I said yes.

3

*And, if we meet, we shall not scape a brawl; For now,
these hot days, is the mad blood stirring.*
William Shakespeare, *Romeo and Juliet*

Funny the way things work out. All part of life's long division,
I suppose.

Having talked me into joining his staff in Ward 25 by
saying I did not need to be a fighter, Charlie made sure the
first thing I did before I set foot on the ward floor was take
part in a Control and Restraint course. I had to learn to
protect myself from aggression and to help restrain violent
individuals safely. That all sounded a lot like being a fighter
to me. Or, at least, being trained to be a fighter 'in case the
need ever arose'. Like a bad whiff from a drain, the first little
doubt as to the wisdom of my decision wafted into my mind.

The course turned out to be not just a day-long thing either;
it consisted of *five* days' theory and practical application.
Monday to Friday; mornings and afternoons; nine till twelve;
one till four. That's a lot of not being a fighter to learn. And
a lot of not being aggressive to handle. The reason for the
depth of the course, I learned the first day, was that the nurse
I was replacing had broken a patient's arm during a restraint.
He hadn't meant to. The patient involved was particularly
aggressive – especially towards him – and had gone berserk
one evening, requiring six big burly men to take him down
and sit on him (metaphorically) until he saw the error of his

ways and agreed to behave. The arm-break had happened purely accidentally, in the course of an unusually prolonged and violent struggle. But still, during the course of a restraint in the ward, a patient's arm had somehow become broken.

The Trust had decided that this was a Bad Thing. Patients having their arms broken during restraints was Not Good Practice. In fact, it was Less Than Satisfactory. It shouldn't happen again, if it could be avoided. The best way to avoid it was to have in-service training. And not just for meek and green newcomers like myself. The entire staff of the ward had to be retrained (or in many cases simply trained) not to break people's arms. The retraining programme took several weeks, a proportion of the ward staff – both day and night personnel – being engaged for five days at a time. Once the period of training was over, no member of staff was to be allowed onto the Locked Ward unless they were trained in C & R. Thereafter, no limbs – patients or staff – should end up being broken, no matter what the situation. This was surely a Good Thing.

The course was held in the rec hall of the old asylum. It was run by a man called Eric who had, at one time, been the charge nurse of the Locked Ward. Eric was in good shape; he obviously worked out. (I, on the other hand, was not in good shape and for some years had obviously worked *in*). Some years previously Eric had seen the need for expert C & R training in various work locations, not just for psychiatric nurses but also other people like air crew, teachers, traffic wardens, correctional facility staff and so on. He knew his stuff.

Each morning we started off by limbering up, to get ourselves 'fit and loose', as Eric said. The second whiff floated through my mind. But it was all part of a properly constructed and modularised course. It all clicked together like Lego.

He started with de-escalation, disengagement and breakaway techniques. De-escalation means exactly that – taking the heat out of a confrontation, appeasing someone mad with rage or resentment, talking softly and soothingly to him. If de-escalation doesn't work, then you move on to disengagement and breakaway – methods of extricating yourself from the grip of the mad person, now intent on visiting harm upon your fragile little body. So, the scenario might go thus:

Mad person: Ah'm gonnae pull your fuckin' head off!
You: Now, now. There's no need to lose your temper. Tell me what you find unsatisfactory or not up to par at the moment.
Mad person: It's Thursday!
You: I agree with you.
Mad person: So ah'm gonnae pull your fuckin' head off.
You: Ah, but it's not my fault that it's Thursday.
Mad person: Naw, but Kylie Minogue's no here, so you'll need tae dae!
You: Let's talk about this.

Then the mad person grabs you in a headlock or tries to choke you, or grabs you by the goolies. There is imminent danger of him pulling your fucking head off. Or your goolies. Neither is a Desirable Outcome. In fact, if your goolies are pulled off, there is little point in anything being desirable again.

Disengagement comes in handy here. Eric showed us techniques for the swift and slippy getting out of holds. Headlock – push his elbow up, slide your head to the side and down – hey presto, you're oot. An attempt to choke – quickly slide your hand lengthwise between his hands and your neck. Step to the side and twist – hey presto again. Grabbed by the goolies – squawk in a very high voice and pee all over his hand. (I may not be remembering all of this with 100 per cent accuracy; it happened some time ago.)

Eric was very impressive. He was lissom, fit and strong. No matter the situation – and he regularly ordered one of the class to attack him with full vigour – he freed himself with balletic skill and dispatch. Then he showed us how to do it. I got quite good at breaking away and disengaging.

By the afternoon of Day 2, however, we were past the foothills of de-escalation and disengagement, and heading for the ridges and crevasses of control and restraint: stopping, controlling and neutralising aggressive incidents. Not fighting, of course. Restraint.

Eric showed us how to engage with a violent patient, disarm him where necessary, render him incapable of further aggression, and remove him from the scene where appropriate. It ended up, in the best examples, with the patient safely restrained, face down, on the floor, with one NA restraining one arm, a second NA the other, and a third NA the legs. In this situation, if performed correctly, the patient's back and chest were unhindered, so that he could breathe, while he was incapable of using his limbs for any aggressive purpose. In this position too it was easy for another member of staff to administer sedative medication if required – usually an injection in the buttock.

As Eric pointed out, it was a considerable responsibility, restraining a person without imposing pain – which was what we were supposed to do. And not break arms, either. Police, for example, were trained differently. They could apply pain until the victim gave up and became biddable. We had to eliminate any threat without harming the aggressor. It made sense. There is a difference between someone who is being aggressive because of an illness, and someone who is being aggressive because he is a bad so-and-so. I saw the force of it all. In fact, I saw the force of quite a lot.

Because the practical section of the course involved working through restraining techniques with colleagues, I gave the assembled throng the old snake eye. At least two of the female nurses were youngish and prettyish. So, getting to grips with either of them would have been an acceptable way of passing an afternoon's control and restraint. Didn't happen.

There were two young, hefty and fit men. I didn't fancy being paired up with either of them. I was paired up with Graeme. Graeme was a big boy. And a broad boy. And a very strong boy. And if that gives the impression that he was three boys, I can assure you there were times when it felt like it. And I bruise like a peach. Trying to escape from quite a few stones of Graeme, when he was straddling my chest and attempting to choke me – purely as an exercise, of course – wasn't a lot of laughs. It was all starting to feel a fair bit like fighting.

But we got to Friday afternoon, and the course came to an end, by which time my body had started to resemble a Dalmatian's. My pasty little white body was now dumplinged with bruises. I got my certificate, though. I was legal. I was C & R trained. I could restrain people without breaking their arms. The next week I would start in the IPCU as an NA.

The night before my first shift in the Locked Ward, I dreamed I was an orderly in a Victorian asylum, with a cage over my head and a truncheon through my belt. The place was gloomy and cold as a dungeon. Naked madmen, with their heads shaved against lice, were chained to the stone walls howling lunatic bans. I paced along a terrace of cells, peering through the grated windows of each door. In a padded room a straitjacketed maniac bounced off the walls. Fellow orderlies, caged and truncheoned, turned a hose on a violent fight between two inmates. In the last room a man was being restrained on an operating table as a surgeon prepared to trepan him. The surgeon placed the point of a chisel on the patient's brow and brought the mallet up to strike . . .

I woke up with my heart going round the drum kit.

4

'But I don't want to go among mad people,' Alice remarked.
'Oh, you can't help that,' said the Cat. 'We're all mad here.
I'm mad. You're mad.'
'How do you know I'm mad?' said Alice.
'You must be,' said the Cat. 'Or you wouldn't have come here.'

Lewis Carroll, *Alice's Adventures in Wonderland*

Thankfully, the ward, when I got there, was nothing like that. It was modern, bright and freshly painted, with plenty of windows admitting light. Unopenable windows, certainly. Of unbreakable glass. But they let the light in.

It was basically an L-shape, the longer leg of the L being the corridor from the entrance to the bedded area, the shorter section at right angles. There was a heavy main door, with a long vertical window of toughened glass, that gave a view up the entire length of the ward. This door was only used in emergencies or to admit beds, trolleys and other large items of furniture. There were two smaller, windowless, interlocking doors on either side of the main one. Each of these could be opened with a key or by means of a swipe card, and gave access to a small vestibule – the Buffer Zone. The outer door was secured, and then the locked inner door was opened – again by key or swipe – onto the ward. Neither door would open until the other was securely closed. This airlock system minimised opportunities for escape and allowed staff to speak to visitors, check bags for forbidden items, and so on.

On entry, the main office was on the left. Here staff did paperwork, answered phones, talked to consultants, junior doctors, visitors and occasional patients. On one wall was a board with a diagram of the ward layout, studded with small lights. Each staff member was given an alarm at the start of the day, a compact device about the size of a mobile phone. In moments of need, a press on the alarm would trigger a loud electronic two-note siren. The light corresponding to your position on the ward lit up. Then everyone free came running to your assistance. Usually. There was another board at the top end of the ward. In moments of *absolute* emergency, when the ward resembled the Ypres Salient, staff could send out a Treble Three. Dialling this told the hospital operator that the Locked Ward needed mucho reinforcements. PDQ. There was a CCTV monitor in the office, and a buzzer/intercom that connected with another at the front door of the unit. So that, whether you called in broad white daylight, or during the tiniest smithereen of the wee small hours, you could communicate with the staff, be seen by them and, possibly, be allowed in.

The door into the courtyard was adjacent to the office. The courtyard had planters full of flowers.

Opposite the office were the Smoke Room and the GP Room, where patients could play music, work with computers or play video games, do artwork of all kinds or take part in group activities. Smoking was prohibited in the hospital, as is generally the case – medical folk tend to have a dim view of the hobby – but not in the psychiatric wards. Smoking was permitted in the room designated for the purpose. The prevailing ethos was still anti – a succession of Smoking Cessation nurses came and went from the ward, attempting to wean patients off the weed – though I thought that it was not the best time to go about it, when people were banged up under all sorts of stress.

Further up the ward was the Charge Nurse's office, where staff meetings and executive decisions took place, and the Off-Duty was made up. The Off-Duty was the paradoxical term used in the hospital for the duty roster. The shift pattern was two days on, two days off – except for weekends, when staff were either on or off duty for the Saturday, Sunday and Monday. Obviously, every second week, staff got a long weekend. It was every first week that was the hassle. Three days on, when everyone else was going out to the cinema, or the match, or the boozer, or anything else for that matter, was purgatory. For me, at least. And it never ceased to be. The fact that the roster was known as the 'Off-Duty' would seem to endorse my view. It was obvious which part of it was most valued by staff.

Opposite the Charge Nurse's office was a small Games Room with a pool table. Very occasionally, during moments of high tension, this would be locked. Pool cues and billiard balls make very effective weapons.

There were two Interview Rooms, where the medical staff could talk to patients, usually with at least one NA present for security. One of these rooms had a phone that patients were allowed to use. Ten, fifteen, twenty times a day we unlocked the door for a patient to make a call, and locked it again as they left. Sometimes we had to monitor their calls. It happened more than once that a patient phoned the police and told them we were holding him prisoner – could they send a squad to release him?

A small corridor after the Pool Room led to the Dayroom, which was split into the dining and TV areas. Meals were served from a hatch in the small pantry-cum-kitchen. Then there was the door through to the bedded area. Each patient had his or her own room, with a bed, a small chest of drawers, a wardrobe, a table and an ensuite toilet/shower room. If necessary, the frame around each door could be dismantled with a screwdriver in slip-jig time. It was not unknown for a patient, in times of extreme distress, to attempt to barricade himself in. Then it might be essential to get to him before he harmed himself. There were twelve bedrooms in all. Also in this area were the Treatment Room, the Laundry Room, the Bathroom and several storerooms, one with a set of twelve boxes fixed to the wall where patients' property could be stored. This was known as the 'Dookits'. Just through the doorway through to the bedded area was a desk and telephone, known as the Nurses' Station. Sometimes, staff smoked here.

For obvious reasons, all glass in doors and windows was toughened. Unbreakable. And the shower rails flipped off the wall if you hung anything as heavy as a regret on them.

(I include this brief functional passage to familiarise the reader with the geography. And also because, on my first morning there, that's precisely what Charlie did for me.)

During the course of this ten-bob tour, some patients paid as little attention to me as if I'd been a snatch of music or a smell of Bisto, while some smiled, said hello and asked my name. One or two – Harriet and Bernard spring to mind – even shook my hand and said they hoped I would be happy working there. It could have been a garden party. If it hadn't been for the young man who now walked into the Dayroom and suddenly bawled into my face, at a blood-curdling level, 'They've killed him! They've fuckin' killed him!'

This was not a settling thing to happen. I failed in spirit rather spectacularly and only just managed not to jump like a cat into Charlie's arms. My blood pressure rocketed and I turned to look at the bearer of this awful news. He was now heading off in the opposite direction.

'My God!' I said to Charlie. My heart was bounding out of my shirt.

'Yeah. That's Gus,' he said. 'He's extremely ill at the minute. Fairly obviously. Needless to say, nobody's murdered anybody. He's not a violent or aggressive man, by any means. Never been involved in anything violent. It's a recurring delusion he has.'

A young woman passed. She was wearing a black sleeveless top and white jeans. Her hair was lying damply against her head and neck, as if she had only then emerged from the shower, and her face was plastered with cold cream. She gave me a brilliant smile, like a White and White Minstrel.

None of the patients in the area had reacted in the slightest to Gus's outburst. In fact, Harriet smiled sympathetically and said, 'Poor Gus.' I saw a female nurse in the corridor put her arm around his shoulder and accompany him towards the Smoke Room.

Charlie had to take a phone call. Since I was not averse myself, in those times, to blackening a lung, I decided to add a few drops of nicotine to my dose for the day. The Smoke Room was a poky little affair. You didn't actually need to light up when you went in. The air itself was enough to kipper your lungs in an instant. It was roughly the size of a linen cupboard and every patient who smoked, which was most of them, had to get their nicotine fix in there. So you can imagine how the clouds rolled by. The atmosphere was similar to that of Uranus. I sparked up and added to the fug.

Besides Gus, there were two younger people in the smoking area. Both were good-looking kids in their late teens or early twenties, one male, one female. The young man, Oliver, smiled – a warm and welcoming one. The young woman, Elaine, smiled also. But there was an edge to her smile. It was no more than a drawing back of her lips. It struck me as the rictus of a predator smelling a fresh victim. Gus sat and stared straight ahead, smoking viciously.

And then the door opened and my arse fell off in fright and rattled on the floor like a hubcap. A tall and powerfully built young man with an extremely intense expression entered. I doubted if anyone had ever kicked sand in his face. If he had ever been a seven-stone weakling, he'd been twelve years old at the time. He had looked after himself. I had not. (You too can have a body like mine. If you spend most of your time on your backside, behind a book.) He had an intimidating walk, most of it propelled by his shoulders, it seemed. Too young to be a silverback, on the street he would still have been an alpha male. But what chilled me was his burning gaze. I had never seen anyone with a look of such intensity. Little did I know I was to meet someone else with an even better one just shortly. The young man looked around. He had an unlit cigarette between the fingers of his right hand

'All right, Archie?' said Elaine.

Archie ignored her.

'New nurse,' Elaine said.

Archie now looked directly at me and moved forward. He stopped in front of me and held his cigarette up to his mouth.

'Got a light?' he growled.

'Sure.' I clicked my lighter and sparked his fag. He took a couple of quick drags, then looked at me again.

'You new?'

'Aye.'

'S your name?'

'Dennis.'

He didn't look impressed by this information. He nodded and walked to a seat by the window, opposite Gus. Elaine and Oliver resumed the conversation I had obviously interrupted, about how she hated her 'fuckin' mother, the bitch'. I ground my stub out in an ashtray and left.

Ward 25 was proving to be interesting, if a little unsettling. Gus's screech and Archie's scorcher had both unsettled me, even if I was soon reassured about both. I had never before encountered anything like them. But that is the source of most people's problems with mental illness. It is the unknown that terrifies us in life, the unfamiliar and the unpredictable. People fear what they're not sure of. What they cannot control. It's *The Old Dark House* again. If we don't know what's in a dark and quiet place, we fill it with bogeymen and demons. Here be dragons.

The lunch trolley came in. At breakfast, lunch and dinner a porter opened the outer door and left a heavy catering trolley in the Buffer Zone. When he exited, the inner door became openable and a member of staff fetched it in. An orderly wheeled it up the corridor now.

Patients started to converge upon the dining area. Elaine and Oliver came up behind me from the Smoke Room. Gus, now noticeably quieter and more guarded in his appearance, arrived. Harriet and Bernard were there. And another patient stood up from a seat by the TV. At the same time John, one of the orderlies, stood up from the seat by him. John had been 'specialing' him. This term meant that, for whatever reason, and there might be many, the patient was accompanied by a staff member at all times. The situation was also known as 'close observation', 'close obs' or just 'close'. They all meant the same thing. Depending on the severity of a patient's condition, the staff member on close might be within walking distance or arm's length. Or the situation might require that two or, rarely, even more staff be on special.

The man who stood up and now approached the hatch in the company of John was stocky, with dark curls and a fleshy face. As he passed, he gave me a murderous stare. Once again I was in danger of misplacing my rump. Nobody here liked me.

The shift I worked with consisted of between ten and twelve people. There was Charlie. There were also John and Luke, very experienced IPCU orderlies who had been in the ward when it was part of the old asylum and had moved with it to Ward 25 in the hospital. They were big and strong and could handle themselves. I liked being around them at the start, for obvious reasons. Clyde was from Jamaica. He had started in a psychie ward in Kingston, done his training, and had gradually drifted away from the Caribbean and in a generally north-easterly direction until he'd settled here. He was tall and athletically built. He played cricket – which West Indian doesn't? – football, basketball and golf. When all of that got dull for him, he ran and boxed. I had no objection to being in his company either. Nor did the ladies. It seemed that his dark skin, athletic build and voice – smooth and sweet as molasses – appealed to them considerably. Clyde thought that the world was accompanied by a constant wave of gentle sound, like the susurration of angel breath. In reality it was just the soft whisper of ladies' eyelashes fluttering whenever he passed by. And there was Gordon, another orderly, who was not the cutest pair of knickers in the drawer. There were always supposed to be three males on the floor at any given time, although sometimes it was not possible. Annual leave, sick leave, in-service training, meal breaks – as in any occupation, any of these could reduce numbers at any time.

There were females on the staff too. Pamela and Geraldine were trained nurses, RNs practised with the soft shoulder and the sympathetic ear, as well as ready with the tablets and deft with injections. There was Ursula, an NA. And there was Rona, an older lady, another NA and something of a mother figure to some of the patients.

Most of these people had worked in the old asylum – in fact, only Clyde, Gordon and myself had not. Their range of experience was invaluable. And very comforting. John explained that Ward 25 was a vast improvement on the asylum IPCU. It was up to date, bright and welcoming; each patient had his or her own room and therefore privacy, and so on. The only downside was that the asylum had been set in beautiful scenic grounds. Trees. Shrubberies. Smooth lawns. Birdsong. In Ward 25, instead of green trees and fresh air, patients had the courtyard, surrounded on all sides by the high walls of the hospital. On good days they got a patch of blue sky. The ward was in the hospital basement. They called it the 'lower ground floor' but it was the basement. A dungeon. An oubliette. That was a pity. It smacked of 'We'll just hide the loonies in the crypt.' I don't suggest for a moment that that was the thinking. It just had that unfortunate zing about it.

Surprisingly perhaps, certainly to a burned-out old hippy of liberal values like myself, the person responsible for the closure of the old asylums was Enoch Powell.

In an address he delivered to the National Association of Mental Health annual conference in 1961, he set out plans to dismantle the huge asylums of previous generations and to embark upon a ten-year programme of general hospital building, and stated that, for the most part, the mentally ill should be treated in 'wards and wings of general hospitals'. And he described the old asylums thus:

'There they stand, isolated, majestic, imperious, brooded over by the gigantic water-tower and chimney combined, rising unmistakable and daunting out of the countryside – the asylums which our forefathers built with such immense solidity to express the notions of their day.' This has become known as the 'Water Tower' speech, and was much more visionary, as well as much less controversial, than his 'Rivers of Blood' one. It's hard not to agree with his analysis of the situation as it was back then, and hard not to see that moving the vast majority of patients into wards of hospitals, where they had the chance and the ultimate goal of rejoining society, was right.

The Victorians built the asylums. The word is Greek, and means shelter or refuge. And that is precisely how the Victorians saw their function: to provide a place of refuge for the insane. As Powell said, most were massive edifices of brick and stone. Many had extensive grounds, as had our old local asylum. Patients, as part of their treatment or therapy, worked in the grounds, trimming lawns and tending shrubberies. Where these things existed, patients also worked in farms, laundries or bakeries attached to the asylums. But there were still straitjackets, padded rooms and restraint chairs. Patients were there for most of their lives in some cases. They became dehumanised. Depersonalised. Institutionalised. The asylums were renamed 'mental hospitals'. An asylum by any other name would smell as hopeless. Far from being refuges, they became castles of despair. Their time was almost come. The 'anti-psychiatry' movement of the 1960s had grave concerns that some treatments did far more damage than good to patients, who were often treated against their will. There was, too, growing humanitarian concern over such vast institutions being unaccountable.

And so they had to go.

_____

5

Your noble son is mad.
Mad call I it. For, to define true madness,
What is't but to be nothing else but mad?
William Shakespeare, *Hamlet*

The working day in Ward 25 was much less onerous and
task-driven than it had been in Care of the Elderly. There
was no waking, washing, shaving, dressing and feeding in the
morning. Patients were simply informed at 8.30 that breakfast
was ready. There was no toileting round. There was no
putting-to-bed ritual in the evening. In that regard it was much
easier work. But there was always the threat of violence.

Gordon the galoot told me in his pompous way that
being an NA in the Locked Ward was a bit like being a
soldier in the trenches in the First World War: there were
long stretches of boredom and occasional flashes of violent
activity. The analogy is not unjust; it's just slightly pompous.
Hence Gordon's galootery.

A typical working day consisted of arriving for work at
7.30 and getting the handover information from the night
staff – any incidents, areas of concern or new admissions.
Then, after a coffee and a knuckle of fags, we served
breakfast. Every door was knocked on, every patient
informed that breakfast was served. In my first few years
there all patients had to be up and vacate the bedded area by
nine o'clock. This area was then locked off until after lunch,

so that the domestic staff could clean the bedrooms and corridors thoroughly. A drug round took place at breakfast. Pick-me-ups and calm-me-downs were handed out, where prescribed, and then staff had their own breakfast. Morning activities followed. There was a visiting hour from eleven till twelve, and lunch was served around 12.15. After lunch the bedded area was opened for two hours, and patients were free to go back to their rooms and sleep, listen to music or just be alone. Staff lunches took place then, at staggered intervals. There was a second visiting hour between two and three o'clock. Dinner was 5.30 and the last visiting hour was from seven till eight. From about six o'clock onwards, on most evenings, we were winding down for handover to the night staff at 8.30 p.m. Clinical notes were written up and all sorts of menial chores – the changing of beds, the bagging and removal of garbage, the putting away of freshly laundered linen – performed. This was the spine of the working day.

In the course of my first days on the ward the patients I met represented, to a significant degree, the complicated range of serious mental illness. Almost all suffered from some kind of psychosis, but one of the most important things I learned from my time there was that there are as many illnesses as there are people. All different. All unique. All requiring to be treated seriously, individually and with delicacy. And now would appear to be as good a time as any to define 'psychosis' and to draw the distinction between that and 'neurosis'. I had no idea what the difference was until I worked there.

Simply put, a neurosis (or, more commonly nowadays, neurotic disorder) is a mental disorder where normal responses to everyday things are exaggerated. The patient may well be distressed, indeed may well suffer – suffer greatly – but they don't lose contact with reality. There are no delusions, no hallucinations. But neurosis is not a minor illness. The fact that the word 'neurotic' is often used loosely outside medical circles might give that impression. It is a wrong impression. People sometimes use 'neurotic' to describe someone they consider flighty, or overly anxious about things. Neurosis is not insignificant. The degree of unhappiness experienced can be crippling. It may have a significant negative impact on day-to-day life. A phobia, for example, is a neurotic disorder. A sufferer may have an exaggerated fear of birds and other flying creatures which may restrict their time outdoors, and any venture out of the house may be full of anxiety.

'Psychosis', literally translated from Greek, means an abnormal condition of the mind and is most commonly associated with loss of contact with reality. Hallucinations, delusional beliefs and thought disorder are common symptoms.

Harriet, who had been so welcoming on my arrival, was a plump woman, maybe in her late forties, with long grey hair that had probably once been fair. She usually pinned it up and fastened it with a barrette and slides, but when she let it down and brushed it out, her hair reached to the small of her back. I suspected she had been vain about it in her youth. Probably with good reason. Her bosom was massive, and her backside likewise. She wore vast tops and floor-length skirts, completely hiding her feet, so that she gave the impression, as she moved majestically up the corridor, that she was on castors.

She turned out to be an extremely pleasant woman, always smiling and trying to be helpful to other people.

And always talking. I mean *always*. ALWAYS. Incessantly. Without remit. Once I was established, she would stop me in the corridor and say, 'Oliver's smoking in there you know smoking is a very bad habit that's well known it's been an established medical fact for over twenty years that it can cause cancer I realise it's a smoking room but he's only young and I don't think he should be ruining his health like that he smokes nonstop chain smoking they call it he lights up a new one from the end of his last of course he'd be perfectly entitled to tell me to mind my own business if I said anything to him because I'm not his mother but I think maybe you could say something Dennis it's not my place you're staff you're a man you seem like a person who knows about these things he might listen to you he's a nice young man but he needs an older man's guidance and I'm sure you're the very man for it. Emphysema's as bad.'

And she'd walk away.

Or she'd take her tray from me at the hatch and say, 'Somebody told me that you should chew your food thirty-two times before you swallow it I don't see how that can be the case if it's a meal like steak or pork or something hard like that or a gammon steak even they're nice with a ring of pineapple on the top then you might be able to chew it thirty-two times with every mouthful but what about pasta that's going to slip down much more easily I think they must mean something harder than that macaroni or spaghetti or what is it you call the twirly ones they've got an Italian name that means twirly they're all different types but they're all basically just pasta not everything is the same texture is it that would just be stupid some things are really soft but others are hard and what about ice cream? Thank you very much.'

And she'd go to her seat.

Or she'd come up to me by the Treatment Room and say, 'Would it be possible for me to have some medication Dennis if you're not too busy I don't mean medication like well you know what I mean I'm only talking about an aspirin I've got a bit of a sore head not a migraine I don't suffer from those thankfully I knew a woman once in our street suffered from the migraine and she was a martyr to it had to lie down in darkened rooms and not go out in the light couldn't see for days well not properly she could see a little probably enough to differentiate between light and shade maybe I don't mean she went blind although I dare say she probably felt like it every time it happened to her she had a terrible time of it four or five times a year she took it I don't mean anything like that I've just got a sore head like anybody gets. Or maybe a paracetamol.'

Now, despite Charlie's initial certainty that I could talk and listen to people, I am not by nature a man for chit-chat. Like Shakespeare's Don John, I am not of many words. Not in speech, at least. I read somewhere that a woman speaks on average 21,000 words a day, whereas a man uses 7,000 – a third of that. You can third that down again for me. I can't be doing with talk for the sake of it. Leave thy vain bibble-babble. No, I'm a real silence-is-golden man. And someone chattering away like a magpie would, in the ordinary course of events, draw a smart rebuke. A real stinger. Empty vessels, and all that. However, I was aware that Harriet was ill, so I made allowances. It's one of my more magnanimous qualities. But I must be honest. There were some days when the smile I managed to scrape onto my face was decidedly wintry, when she accosted me for the fourth time in half an hour to give me one of her Molly Bloom soliloquies.

Harriet's garrulity wasn't necessarily a symptom of her illness. Or a product of it. At least one staff colleague – Gordon – had even more stickability in his tongue than she did. He was a real stayer when he was in the mood. No donkeys had hind legs anywhere in his vicinity. His tongue must have been glad when he went to sleep. Gordon is the only human being I've ever come across whose conversation had automatic resumption, like the iPlayer. It didn't matter how long it was since you last saw him, he would resume the conversation you were last having, as if you'd just got up to shut the window because there was a draught.

One day he was telling me at toe-curling length about how his next-door neighbour had bought a pup for the youngest one's birthday. A common symptom among talkers like Gordon is that they can't read the signals that their listener has lost interest – if he ever had any. Yawns, shifting of position in one's chair, looking in the other direction – all to no avail. Even falling asleep or feigning sudden death have no effect. Despite my many sighs, bum shuffles and the occasional whimper of helplessness; despite the fact that I got up twice to go to the lavatory in the middle of it all, on he ploughed. I heard about the child's age, how she was awfully clever, how her parents had arrived at her name – a tortuous process in itself – why they decided on a dog as a present, and much, *much* more. I considered just leaving and having a shave at one point.

Then Charlie told him to go for lunch. How my old heart sang. After the hour that took, I had my own lunch break. So it was well over two hours before he saw me again. In the meantime he had driven home and had a conversation over lunch with his flatmate; I had gone for a listen to my iPod and a sleep in the GP Room, and various other weighty matters had occurred. I took over close obs from John at a patient's door and Gordon appeared at my shoulder.

'Onyhoo,' he said, 'it's wan a they Labradoodles. They've called it Toby.'

And we have gobshites aplenty on every street in the country. Some people love to talk. It's just that I don't. But Harriet was a warm and caring person, and I liked her.

What I didn't know, my first day, was that both Harriet and Bernard were rapidly approaching the time when they could be discharged from the ward. They were 99 per cent well again. Their sojourn in the IPCU, the nursing interventions and the regimen of medication had brought them back up to speed, and soon they would return to society. I never saw Harriet again after she was discharged. She headed back to the delights of wherever she came from and for all I know – and hope – she is still there, burbling away to any passing wedding guest she chances upon, and as happy as a pig in shit.

Bernard was a tall man with a magnificent head of grey hair that he combed in scholarly sweeps down past his ears to his collar and a Jimmy Edwards moustache. And he was intelligent, articulate, polite and solicitous of everyone's well-being. He too was soon for the great outdoors. The next time he was admitted, however, six or seven months into the future, he managed to find a screwdriver, unscrew an ultra-flat brushed-steel socket from the skirting board in a quiet nook of the bedded area, and insert some thin strips of metal into the gubbins of the system, thereby blowing the entire electrics of the ward for a period of three hours. And still, when apprehended for the felony, he maintained his genteel and thoughtful persona.

'I was concerned for the patients, Dennis. Too much electricity can weaken your chances of fatherhood.'

6

His drawers were of rabbit skins; so were his shoes; —
His stockings were skins but it is not known whose; —
His waistcoat and trousers were made of pork chops; —
His buttons were jujubes and chocolate drops . . .

Edward Lear, *The New Vestments*

If 'neurotic' is a term that has been adopted by people outside psychiatry and used loosely, and usually incorrectly, so much more so has the term 'paranoid'. It doesn't just mean 'very suspicious'; it is a symptom, or an element, that can be present in over eighty medical conditions.

Grace was a woman in her forties and, when I knew her, was extremely paranoid. She was mistrustful of staff, particularly new members like myself, and watched us like a bird of prey as we made coffee, served meals or administered medication. If I was on the Cuppa Detail, she would insist that I hand over the jar of coffee for her to scoop her spoonful into her cup, and a similar process went on with the sugar bowl. She couldn't actually pour the hot water herself, because the urn was, for obvious reasons of safety, situated well away from the hatch, but she craned through the hatch and watched as I did it. Then she insisted on taking the carton of milk and pouring her own helping.

She did not speak to me for many days. When she first did, I got quite a turn. I came into the ward at 7.30 one morning to find her just inside the inner door.

'Hello,' she said.

'Hello, Grace. How are you?'

'Your car is the black Nissan, isn't it?' And she reeled off my registration.

'Er, yes,' I replied, a curious sinking sensation in my stomach. 'Why?'

'I just like to know these things. I've been watching you park it.'

'Oh right. Excuse me, Grace. I need to get into the ward and get my coat off.'

She stood back and allowed me to pass. When I emerged from the changing room, she was there again.

'Your name's Dennis, isn't it?'

'It is, aye.'

'What's your second name?'

'Why d'you want to know?'

'Might be useful. Where do you live? I mean, what street? I know the town.'

What creepiness was this? Why the hell did she want to know my name, my address and what kind of car I drove? She didn't look like the kind of person who would stalk somebody but what did I know? I'd been on the ward a handful of shifts. I knew comparatively little about serious mental illness. But I had seen *Play Misty for Me*. Oh Christ, and *Fatal Attraction*! If I divulged any more information, would she wait till she was discharged, then come and get me some night, her face blacked like a commando? Shin up a drainpipe after wringing the necks of a few pigeons to get herself in the mood, and then bludgeon me to death with a knobkerrie? I may have missed the irony at the time, but at this point I was considerably more paranoid than Grace. And if I *had* seen the whimsy of it, I doubt if I'd have laughed much.

I excused myself sharpish saying I had to be present for the overnight report. After Charlie had given us it, I hung back to tell him of my encounter with Grace.

'I mean, she was asking me all these things. Why was she doing that?'

'She's ill, Dennis.'

'Yeah, sure, I know. But what would she do with the information?'

'Nothing. She asks everybody that kind of question. She has a paranoid delusion. It makes her do things like that. She'll get better. And then she won't give a tuppenny fuck about who *you* are or where you live.'

Reassured, I left the office. Grace was coming down the corridor.

'I know where you live,' she said. 'Ursula told me.'

My arse making buttons, I stalked off up the corridor and found Ursula. She was in conversation with John and Rona.

'Did you tell Grace where I live?' I squeaked.

'No,' said Ursula. 'Take a tablet, for God's sake.'

Grace had asked Ursula all right, but Ursula had only mentioned the town, something which Grace already knew but treated as if it were new and valuable information. I did calm down eventually but I was as jittery as a rabbit about it all day. And if I could feel that way about something I knew the reason for, how much worse must it feel to people who suffer persecutory delusions – inexplicable to them but as real as the air they breathe?

I spoke to Grace a day or two before she was discharged. Her condition had improved immensely. She was now my best pal, I suspect because my wife had the same name as her mother. What a difference a few weeks make!

Before, I was terrified of her dropping down my chimney; now we were exchanging personal information like female characters in a Victorian novel. I asked her what it had been like, when she was ill. Did she know she was becoming ill? That she was paranoid?

She said that she could not tell when it was going to happen, and didn't like to fret about it before it did. 'There is no point in meeting trouble halfway, Dennis. It will always go out of its way to meet *you*. Better just deal with things when they arise.'

A sound philosophy. One that I have taken to heart since. Philosophers are not only found sitting around in Greek ruins.

Sometimes, Grace said, she couldn't be sure when she *had* become ill. But she described one experience that brought home forcibly to me some of the distress that she underwent. She told me that, just before her current admission, she had been walking along her own street, a quiet suburban one, when a car passed with a noisy exhaust. To her, the noise of the exhaust was a low, constant, mocking sneer – Ha! Ha! Ha! Ha! Ha! Ha! Ha! – and she knew it was taunting *her*.

Her account was vivid and convincing and very, very frightening. I was given the smallest and most rapid insight into what she had to put up with. I marvelled at her bravery in dealing with such things and her strength in being able to come back from it.

On the Friday of my first week I met a patient who had one of the most florid presentations that I ever came across in all the seven and a half years I worked in Ward 25. 'Florid' in this context means 'fully developed', having the complete set of symptoms associated with a condition. Bill was florid all right. As florid as Kew Gardens. When I first met him, he was not an inpatient. He came every other Friday afternoon, to have his depot injection administered by Charlie, the only nurse he fully trusted. A depot injection is a jab of some medication that is released slowly and consistently into the body over a period of time – in Bill's case, a fortnight.

At about two o'clock that Friday, the outside door buzzer sounded while Luke and I were in the office. Luke checked the monitor and pressed the intercom.

'Come in, Bill,' he said. Then he pressed the door release and said to me, 'Wait till you meet this guy.'

Bill entered the ward dressed in a black jacket. From beneath it some unidentified garment's striped and fringed hem hung like the tallith of an Orthodox Jew. Ludicrously tight drainpipe trousers gave him a look of Max Wall about the legs. He also sported a shapeless black item of headgear with no brim, but with a length of some gauzy material like crêpe de Chine wound around it and flowing down his back in two colourful streams. He had wide burning eyes and, on this occasion, a mad grin. But I always thought this was for effect. Mad as the moon, he nonetheless knew what kind of impression he cut, and often played up to it. He was the most singular individual I had met in my life. Up to that time. I was to meet several candidates for the post over the next wee while.

'Hi, Fred,' he said to Luke. 'Charlie in?'

'Yeah. Just come up to the Treatment Room, Bill. He's in there. Got your stuff drawn up.'

Then Bill got his eyes on me. He rolled them once or twice and grinned.

'New meat, Fred? Who's the new meat?'

'This is Dennis,' said Luke.

'Hmmmm . . .' mused Bill and gave me another capacious wide-mouthed grin.

We walked him up to the Treatment Room, where Charlie greeted him like a friend.

'Hello, Bill. Good to see you.'

'Hi, Charlie. You tae. Where's Fuck Features?'

'Fuck Features' was Dr Marjorie Bankstreet, head consultant in psychiatry and with responsibility for Ward 25. She was a tall slim ascetic-looking woman and Bill's special bête noire. In his eyes she was responsible for his being banged up on a regular basis. Hence 'Fuck Features'. He had one or two other complimentary names for her too. But delicacy forbids. Charlie was perfectly easy with spiking Bill on his own, so Luke and I ghosted. While Charlie was giving Bill his depot in the Treatment Room, I asked Luke about him.

'Why does he call you Fred?'

'Fuck knows,' said Luke. 'He does that with everybody except Charlie. Calls them something else.'

'Weird.'

'Weird as,' confirmed Luke. 'Insists Charlie gives him his depot in the arm. Most folk take it in the buttock because you've got plenty meat there. Not so sore. Not Bill. Thinks that's a bit gay. More manly to take it in the arm like a flu jag.'

For some months this was how and when I met Bill. He was compliant with the depot medication, pitching up at the ward every fortnight to get his jag – only from Charlie – and most times dressed like he had run through a theatrical costumiers in Velcro underwear.

7

O the mind, mind has mountains: cliffs of fall
Frightful, sheer, no-man-fathomed. Hold them cheap
May who ne'er hung there.

Gerard Manley Hopkins, 'No worst, there is none'

If any mental illness has the power to unsettle and cause fear in the general public, it is schizophrenia. The symptoms displayed by many sufferers from schizophrenia are precisely what Joe Public imagines constitute madness, the kind of madness that he sees in movies and reads about in novels. That many schizophrenics have retreated into a world of their own, with little obvious connection to reality, an often disturbing world of scrambled thoughts and hallucinations, a world with its own laws and dimensions, would seem to many to be the ultimate picture of madness. The condition is also, frequently but inaccurately, associated with a high risk of violence. A series of high-profile newspaper articles in recent years, detailing murders and attempted murders committed in the UK by paranoid schizophrenics, has stoked the fires of public imaginings, so that the mere term inspires fear and dread. In fact, most schizophrenics are not violent. Where there is any aggression, it is often turned inward upon the sufferer and emerges as self-harm or suicide attempts.

Before I give an outline of what schizophrenia is, let me first underline what is it not. It's unfortunate that the term comes from two Greek words that mean 'split' and 'mind'.

Unfortunate, because that it is almost precisely what it is not. It is not the classic split personality of popular imagination, the archetypal Jekyll-and-Hyde division of one mind into two different personalities, each quite distinct from the other. Everyone knows the image of a scientist drinking off a potion from a bubbling test tube before turning into his physically deformed and morally repulsive alter ego. It makes good fiction. It does not make good fact.

Nor is it what schizophrenia sufferers experience. Rather than a *split* personality, they often experience a fragmenting or a disintegration of the personality. One patient described it to me as a 'broken mirror' version of himself. He meant that the image of himself that he had always had was still there, but when he was ill the parts were distorted and changed in their focus, not in the places where they ought to be. He could recognise a part of his personality as being his, but it seemed separate from the rest of him, like seeing an eye in a shard of mirror, knowing it was his but not seeing the rest of his face with it.

'Schizophrenia' is actually an umbrella term that psychiatrists use to describe severe mental illnesses which might cause a patient to hear voices, suffer paranoid delusions and hallucinate. This is all extremely frightening and unsettling for the sufferer and may lead to bizarre behaviour and utterances. However, it can affect people in as many different ways as there are sufferers. Some may withdraw into themselves, become guarded in their manner and suspicious of others.

It usually begins in adolescence or early maturity, tends to occur earlier in males than females by about five years on average, but affects both sexes equally. After the first episode, it often recurs and can develop into a long-term disability. Some sufferers recover within five years. Most develop the kind of condition that comes and goes over years and even decades. A few develop a severe, abiding and long-lasting condition.

There is no lab test for the illness and it can only be diagnosed from observation of symptoms. These are divided into positive and negative. Negative symptoms include apathy and being withdrawn, inappropriate moods, blunted emotional response, aimlessness and lack of energy or willpower. Some cases may restrict themselves to simply these symptoms, without any obvious psychosis (as in 'simple schizophrenia'), so that the sufferer is often just considered odd, especially in adolescence. Positive symptoms include hallucinations, delusions and disordered thought processes and perception.

It can be terrifying for the sufferer. Some believe thoughts are being inserted into their minds by an outside agency, often divine or extra-terrestrial. Bill, when he was on the ward, would never watch TV or listen to a radio, precisely because he thought they were putting thoughts into his mind. If he entered the Smoke Room and someone was playing a radio, he'd leave and smoke outside in the yard. Occasionally, the reverse is experienced and the patient feels that his or her thoughts are being extracted from his mind against his will and broadcast aloud. One woman became very upset when the TV appeared to her to be amplifying her thoughts and making them known to everyone in the Dayroom. Voices inside the sufferer's head can provide a sneering and sarcastic commentary on behaviour, or discuss the sufferer. Sometimes, they become command hallucinations, ordering the sufferer to harm himself or somebody else.

Delusions of being under some other person's control are common. One patient in Ward 25 would not let me draw the Dayroom curtains in the morning because she was terrified that the sun's heat would draw her upwards and out of her body. Other beliefs are frequently encountered, such as what the layman would call 'delusions of grandeur', i.e. that the sufferer is God or a monarch, or some celebrity in the public eye. One young woman wrote so many letters to the prime minister, claiming to be his son's abandoned fiancée and threatening dire consequences if she was not immediately reinstated in his love, that the police, possibly tipped off by MI5, called to find out what was going on.

Some believe that they have paranormal powers.

As if all these were not enough, schizophrenics may also suffer from anxiety or depression. Once in a while, staff would come across a patient with very obvious breaks in his train of thought, resulting in speech that had become incomprehensible, through incoherence, abrupt changes of subject or making up completely new words. Bill often displayed symptoms like echolalia (repeating what was said to him) and schizophasia or 'word salad' (uttering disconnected jumbles of words).

For example, Luke might say to him, 'Bill, can you come to the Treatment Room for your depot?'

Bill's reply might be echolalia: 'Can you come to the Treatment Room? Can you? Ha ha. Can I come to the Treatment Room? Come to the Treatment Room? Okay, I'll come to the Treatment Room.' And then he would sing the word depot like a clock ringing the quarters with Westminster chimes: 'Depot, depot, depot, depot; depot, depot . . .'

Or it might be schizophasia: '. . . when you see you beside you, go faraway not so near with, I can see the treatment in the room, if you treat me if you come to me, with you beside, I don't like a treat in a room . . .'

Something else that Bill did, which I never saw in any other patient, was produce a rhyming monologue based on something someone had said to him. Sometimes it was strangely impressive, like a slightly skewed version of a rap. One afternoon I was filling out patients' menus for the next day's meals. Some patients preferred to fill out their own; some couldn't be bothered and preferred you to do it for them. One of the latter was Bill. I asked him, as he glided out of the Dayroom, what he would like for dinner.

'Dinner,' he said, as he slid past me, 'that's a winner. Dinner dinner, you don't eat it, you get thinner. Skinny skinner. Then you fast. Not so fat, not so fast, it won't last.' Halfway down the corridor, he shouted back, 'What is there?'

'Erm, there's cottage pie, fishcakes . . .'

'Cottage pie, that's for me; give it a try, I say aye; chips an' peas, that's for me . . .' And his voice trailed away as he entered the Smoke Room. It might not have been exactly that; I didn't commit it to memory, although I was immensely entertained by it then. He could keep it up for minutes at a time. I ticked the boxes for cottage pie, chips and peas.

What causes schizophrenia is still not completely known but a number of factors have been identified which may affect it: genetic, biochemical and neurochemical, social and psychological. And the term 'schizophrenia' itself is a broad one, covering a wide variety of conditions. It may be acute but short in duration, such as a schizophrenic reaction to an incident, or incidents, of severe stress. Equally, it may be the onset of a longer-term and progressive illness. Several main types have been identified.

'Simple schizophrenia' is marked by odd conduct and an inability to cope in society. It is characterised by the negative symptoms associated with schizophrenia, and is less obviously psychotic than other forms. What often happens is that sufferers become increasingly removed from, or rejected by, society, and end up as vagrants. 'Hebephrenic schizophrenia' (or 'hebephrenia') most commonly starts at puberty and is marked by listlessness, lack of motivation, auditory hallucinations and peculiar mannerisms. Behaviour is often thought to be shallow, silly or immature, with exaggerated emotional responses. Giggling with little reason is common, and speech may be hard to understand. 'Catatonic schizophrenia' is commoner among females and has become rare in the UK over recent years, giving rise to the possibility that many of its typical symptoms were a direct result of institutionalisation. These symptoms include hyperactivity, often alternating with periods of trance-like stupor, hallucinations and bizarre posturing. Patients often hold rigid poses for long periods of time and show no reaction to external stimuli. 'Paranoid schizophrenia', the most common form, is characterised by long-lasting delusions of persecution, usually combined with auditory hallucinations. Consequently, hostility *may* be displayed and the patient may be violent and aggressive towards others. There are other forms of the illness, but these are the most common. There are also what are called 'schizo-affective disorders', in which the symptoms of mania (or sometimes depression) are co-present with the distortion of perception that is typical of schizophrenia.

Why schizophrenia disturbs carers and loved ones so much is that it appears to destroy the sufferer's personality and ability to live in the real world. One of the most distressing things about it is the social isolation that can result, with patients unable to work, or relate to friends and family. Problems can be complicated and magnified by the way workmates, friends or family respond, especially if they talk slightingly or judgementally.

Treatment consists of different elements – physical, psychological and social. Back in the day, when the illness was not fully understood, patients were subjected to the cruellest procedures including bleeding, leeching, cupping, immersion in cold water, the injection of all manner of unlikely cures, electroconvulsive therapy and insulin-induced comas. Genuine and prolonged relief from symptoms of schizophrenia only came with the development of antipsychotic medication.

Once a patient is discharged from hospital, the support of other people is vital. Social, recreational and occupational therapies are important in helping the patient gain motivation and confidence. GPs, community nurses, social workers, hobbies and special interest clubs all contribute to the gradual rebuilding of a patient's identity. But no group or person is more important than the patient's family or friends – his loved ones.

It's not easy caring for and supporting someone with a major illness like schizophrenia, but there are groups and agencies with the expert knowledge needed to help. People may find that communication with the sufferer will change. The patient's behaviour may change too, becoming more difficult. There will be regular stressful situations, and the sufferer as well as the carer may find it very difficult to deal with these. It's important to take time and effort to find out what works. People are people, with all their differences and personal preferences. The fact that someone suffers from schizophrenia does not alter that. Some patients will appreciate a great deal of direct help; others will resent it as interference. But people respond best to people. There's a lot to learn about the individual patient's preferences. And a lot of readjustment might be necessary. For example, criticisms that seem small in normal family situations may be taken as a huge insult by a person suffering from schizophrenia. Paradoxically, caring too much can seem like intrusion.

The best thing any carer can do is learn about the illness first – what to expect and, perhaps as important, what not to expect. Then the carer can help increase the patient's independence: encourage the sufferer to take an interest, do his or her own washing and shopping, cook where practicable, perform the countless little tasks and chores that go to make up daily life.

The positive thing about schizophrenia nowadays is that sufferers, with very few exceptions, can look forward to spending much of their time, if not most of it, out of locked wards and psychiatric hospitals. Once they would have been incarcerated in asylums for most of their lives. Now, with input from a variety of supporting bodies, they can stay out of them. A consummation devoutly to be wished.

8

His worst fault is, that he is given to prayer;
he is something peevish that way . . .
William Shakespeare, *The Merry Wives of Windsor*

The man with the fell glare being specialed on my first day was called Donnie. That's not enough to make a man glare, in the normal run of things; it's just a fact, a snippet of information I share with you.

Donnie was a big stocky Aberdonian in his mid-twenties, with a head of dark curls and a round face. So far as looks went, he might have been Dylan Thomas, just awake after sleeping off a three-nighter. Or conceivably Brendan Behan, after something similar. The irony of the comparisons is that Donnie never touched a drop. Never had.

His diagnosis was paranoid schizophrenia, but that tells you little about him. He was, in fact, a religious maniac. A complete cake of Religious Fruit and Nut. For him, as for so many, Scripture was not to be interpreted metaphorically. It was all God's truth. Literal truth. God made the world in seven days. Lucifer rebelled and was hurled headlong from heaven into hell, since when he has wandered the world, trying to snare innocent souls to join him in those agonies of the damned. And the agonies of the damned are not the modernistic reading – being without the love of God. We're talking about fire. Eternal, unwavering, everlasting fire. And stench and corruption. In the company of the Devil.

He believed in Christ and the Resurrection too. But in Donnie's faith there was none of the love of the baby Jesus or the benign understanding and forgiveness of any proto-hippy sandalled saviour in a kaftan. It was all fire and brimstone. Sulphur and flames. The wrathful, frogs-and-boils, fiery-furnace God of the Old Testament. Yahweh and the Tales of the Tribes had turned his wits inside out.

When I joined the ward staff, he was brooding and watchful, spending most of his waking time in an armchair by the TV. A male orderly was assigned to be in his vicinity at all times. His look was penetrating and savage enough to punch a hole in someone. He could tell that, beneath the modern clothes and pasty body, I was really the Brute Beast, a lieutenant of the Archfiend, plotting to tip his righteous soul upside down and send it on a chute to Pandemonium. That first day, in the TV Room, I smiled amicably at him. Then I clocked his gimlet stare. Only the woman who does my laundry will know how scared I was. There was a reason for a guy being with him round the clock, and it wasn't in case he got the urge to play dominoes.

This was him on the mend, or so I was reliably informed. In the months before my arrival he had been admitted to the ward after launching himself off a bridge in a transport of religious ecstasy. He had not ascended directly into heaven – much to his disappointment. Instead, he had fallen like a stone, a religious stone, onto the motorway below – thankfully, empty of traffic. Otherwise, he might have achieved martyrdom under the wheels of a truck heading south. Instead, he merely shattered his legs like blackboard chalk. He was pinned together in one of the big hospitals in the city, and walked for a while on crutches.

After this, he was as mad as a snipped snake – partly, no doubt, because he hadn't achieved Glory, but also simply because the whole episode exacerbated his condition. When he had recovered sufficiently to walk again, he made an assault on a nurse in the General Ward and was transferred out to us in the Locked Ward. He had to be placed on close obs, because of his violence and aggression. He would skulk in corners and spring out like a panther at a passing NA, wrestling him to the ground and hissing Scripture. A few incidents like this and he was specialed. Any recurrence meant he would be restrained and jagged.

Much of his hatred and aggression was directed towards himself. One morning Luke was specialing him. Donnie got up, showered, then dressed, all under Luke's supervision. Before heading out for breakfast, he combed his hair in front of the mirror above the handbasin. Luke dallied in his room, allowing him a foot or two of leeway. Out of humane consideration. It must be pleasant, if you're being specialed, to get a slight easing of the screw. Besides, what harm can anybody come to, combing their hair?

John passed by in the corridor, knocking on doors and summoning the faithful to breakfast. Donnie's room door was open.

'The man up, Luke?'

Luke, hands in pockets, looked up.

'Just coming.'

The exchange lasted no more than two seconds.

In those two seconds Donnie had begun to smash his face on the taps in the sink: a rapid and berserk pounding. The noise was appalling: dull fleshy thuds against the metal of the taps. Blood sprayed up the wall and mirror as Donnie's head flicked it around.

Luke dived in to stop him, shouted, 'For fucksake! John!' for assistance and the two men managed to tear him away.

The whole drama had lasted no more than five seconds altogether, but in that time Donnie had inflicted hideous wounds on himself. His face was a soggy mess of blood and torn flesh. He was croaking incoherently, a deep resonant rasp of terror and affliction. And he was struggling wildly.

The mirror had a slash of blood droplets across it. The wall likewise. The sink was spattered with red. Thick blobs of dark blood quivered on the white porcelain.

The guys had to wrestle him to the floor and restrain him. One of them set off his alarm and more staff came running. Two more men joined in the restraint till one of the girls drew a jag up and injected him with the old Relaxy-Voo. Even after being spiked, he struggled violently for quarter of an hour. It took the four men to hold him down all that time.

When they eventually cleaned him up, Donnie's face looked like a Spot-the-Ball entry. He had huge Xs dug into his forehead and his cheeks. The flesh flapped off his face. Swellings and lacerations were starting to blacken up. He was a sorry sight entirely. He would need surgery to sew him back together again.

He did it because he saw the Devil looking back at him out of the mirror.

He had to go to theatre to be patched up. He was given more sedation. John and Luke were to escort him as he was wheeled there on a hospital trolley. A spry wee porter with a bright and cheery disposition arrived at the main door with the wheels. The ward staff helped Donnie to lie down. Helped him quite persuasively.

'And who is this I'm chauffeuring today?' breezed the porter.

'Donnie,' answered Luke.

'Donnie!' enthused the porter.

'The Lord thy God is a jealous God!' growled Donnie from his supine position on the trolley.

'Oh right!' giggled the porter. 'I'll mind that!'

'The Lord. Thy God. Is a jealous God.' Donnie's voice had slowed down and dropped several tones. He was serious.

'Aye!' guffawed the porter.

'He shall cast them into a furnace of fire; there shall be wailing and gnashing of teeth!'

The spry wee porter stopped guffawing as Donnie surged off the trolley, grabbed him by the throat and started to throttle him. Spry no longer, if the wee man had been capable of it by then, he would most certainly have been wailing and even gnashing a tooth or two. His face was magenta and he had the eyes of a tree frog by the time Luke and John tore Donnie's hands from him. More of the old jaggers for Donnie. But he did get patched up.

By the time I arrived in the Locked Ward, his face had healed and he had been on a course of clozapine, an antipsychotic, for several weeks. He had quietened down considerably. Not so considerably that there wasn't still a male orderly in his vicinity at all times, though. Charlie was a thoroughly seasoned Charge Nurse and knew how randomly and impetuously things could change. Luke and John warned me about Donnie, said he was still worth being wary of. After my first encounter with him, I was wary all right. I wore my wary on my sleeve.

Religious concepts are so awe-inspiring and the implications of wrongdoing so overwhelming, it's a wonder not all believers are gibbering wrecks. I'm not one for mysticism or the supernatural, but, as a child, I believed. I believed in all that God and the Devil, heaven and hell, angels and demons stuff. And it makes a profound impression on the childish mind. It's easy to believe in black and white, goodies and baddies, rewarding the good and punishing the bad. Adults tell you this stuff, and they are older and meant to be wiser than you. How can you not love God, when he's done so much for you? How can you not hate the Devil, when he means so much harm towards you? Unfortunately, these concepts burn themselves into the childish mind and prove extremely difficult to erase in later life.

And they drive some people mad.

9

This would be the best of all possible worlds,
if there were no religion in it.

John Adams

John didn't tell me till later, but on my first day in the ward, before I smiled hopefully at him, Donnie had given me the eyeball from his armchair by the TV, then asked John, 'Who's the new nurse?'

'Oh that's Dennis,' John had said. 'You'll like him. He's an old pal of Charlie's.'

Donnie had scrutinised me for a minute or so.

'No. Don't like the look of him at all,' he'd said.

But I grew on him. Like a wart. Certainly, he viewed me at first with as much distaste as if I *had* been visited upon him. No doubt the taint of Belial was about me and he could smell that. For the first few days I worked in 25, if I came into his sight, he'd run me through with that savage glare. He started to speak to me, very grudgingly and suspiciously at first. Very guardedly, he would reply when I asked him whether he wanted tea or coffee, for example. At the hatch, as Grace had done, he would scrutinise my actions carefully: watch very closely which cup I used for him, how I poured the tea from the pot, how I added milk. Everything had to be done in his sight line. Sometimes he would refuse to take the cup I had picked up and would growl, 'Not that one.' Then indicate another. Entirely randomly, it seemed. But then maybe he could see things in the cup that I couldn't.

When I proffered him his dinner tray, I hadn't to lift the metal covers from his dishes. For fear of polluting them. He had to lift each cover himself. He would do so with male staff hovering in the background. Most often he would wrinkle his nose and say, 'No.' Then walk away and leave it. But increasingly often, he would accept, grudgingly, the offered meal and consume at least some of it.

I specialed him for the first time one evening after dinner, about an hour after his evening meds – when he was reckoned to be at his most sedate and mellow. Everything's relative, of course. I sat next to him by the TV, with John and Luke not too far away in the background. For a time he pretended to watch *Corrie*, or something equally uplifting, but I was aware that, although he was facing the screen, he was directing sharp, sideways looks at me. He did this so much he must have had the peripheral vision of a bottle-nosed dolphin. I wasn't at my most relaxed. But I tried some small talk.

'You like *Corrie*, Donnie?'

'*What?*'

He looked at me as if I'd suggested sniffing each other's underwear.

'*Coronation Street*. Do you enjoy it?'

'No.'

'Would you rather I changed the channel?'

'No.'

'Do you watch a lot of TV?'

'No.'

He was so uncomfortable with the conversation that I let him get back to facing the screen and trying to watch me out of his ear. The rest of my spell on watch passed in edgy silence, but without further incident, and then John took over.

The next time I specialed him, he was not quite so antsy. He managed to look ahead and say yes when I asked him if he wanted a cup of tea and a Hobnob. From there, he got to answering my questions when I specialed him in the evenings by the TV. There was a World Cup on that year, and he watched the football. Gradually, he let slip information. He supported Aberdeen. Didn't like Rangers or Celtic. Didn't like any other team. Which meant he suspected they were doctrinally unsound in some way. Didn't know why he was here, couldn't remember how he got here. Led astray by the Devil, probably.

John was sitting at Donnie's room door one afternoon, on close obs, while Donnie sat on his chair and read his Bible. He had an old leather-bound copy, well thumbed, which he spent most of his day reading. This was the only time he ever seemed fully relaxed. The gentle activity of the ward went on around his room. Patients and staff passed; meds were given out; the domestic staff trundled their wheeled mop buckets up the ward; and Luke paced down it on sentry-go. Donnie was quiet.

Ursula came breezing in, in her customary way, still with her coat on and bringing the freshness of the outside air with her. She had a plastic carrier in each hand. She had been out to the shops and had fetched back some purchases for the patients. Fags was a standard request. Sweets. Magazines. Sometimes somebody took a hankering for a vanilla-iced doughnut or a tub of popcorn, maybe a steak and onion bridie – the sort of thing that was difficult to source within the hospital itself. Often staff who were going out at lunchtime made the effort to shop for punters who were not allowed time out.

Ursula clipped about, busily handing out messages and change to this one and that. One girl, Carrie, complained that Ursula had got her the wrong brand of something, I can't remember what. Ursula pointed out that the brand she wanted hadn't been available. Carrie said she should have gone to another shop. Ursula said she hadn't had time; it was her lunch break and she was doing her a favour. Carrie asked Ursula snottily if she was casting it up. Ursula said no, but she hadn't had much time, so she got the next best thing. And if Carrie didn't like it, too bad. Carrie eventually took the item with pretty poor grace and shut her door.

'God almighty!' Ursula snapped.

Suddenly Donnie was at his doorway, brandishing his Bible, eyes blazing.

'Thou shalt not take the name of the Lord thy God in vain!' he roared.

'Cool it, Donnie,' said John, standing up rapidly. 'Ursula didn't mean anything.'

'Are you mocking me for reading the Bible?'

'Not at all,' said John, bracing himself. 'Not at all. I said nothing. Ursula was just frustrated.'

'The Lord will not hold him guiltless that taketh his name in vain.'

'We get the point,' said John.

'I'm sorry, Donnie,' said Ursula, trying to make light of the matter. 'Carrie annoyed me. She was just so ungrateful. I shouldn't have said it.'

Donnie turned the heat in his eyes down from blazing to just wild. He favoured Ursula with a withering glance.

'Idolator,' he sneered. 'Papist. Worshipper of the Beast.'

He turned on his heel and stalked imperiously back to his chair and his reading.

'Well,' said John. 'That's you tellt.'

'And me no even a Catholic,' wondered Ursula as she clipped away to take her coat off.

Slowly, very slowly, as slowly as continental drift, Donnie got used to me. I don't claim that he got to like me, or to trust me, but he grew accustomed to my face and seemed to resent it less. So much so that, when it came time to take Donnie out of the ward, Charlie asked me to escort him up to the canteen on the top floor of the hospital and let him buy himself a meal.

Charlie was one of those Charge Nurses who wouldn't ask you to do what he hadn't done himself. When guys like Donnie became eligible for time out, usually on escorted passes initially, Charlie always did the first escort or two. Donnie had been out around the grounds with him twice and had neither bitten the heads off crows nor called down the wrath of God upon idolators. When Charlie suggested he might now enjoy a stroll to the dining room upstairs and the chance to purchase himself a meal on his next time out, Donnie had agreed. Then he had requested my presence as his escort.

'Me? He asked for me?' I said. I was sitting in the office, facing Charlie across his desk as he wrote notes.

'Aye. You. He asked for you,' Charlie said, writing.

'Specifically?'

Charlie looked up.

'No, not specifically. He asked for any nurse we had who was small, balding, bearded and with a degree in English. You're the only one that fits the bill.'

Sometimes Charlie's wit was as dry as dog biscuits. I looked at him. He smirked and went back to his writing.

'Aye, you specifically,' he chuckled. 'He specified you. Dennis, he said.'

'I thought he didn't like me.'

'How wrong can you be?' Charlie smirked again. 'It's just like *Pride and Prejudice*, isn't it?'

'Okay.'

'Take him when everybody else has had theirs.'

'Right. You sure this'll be all right?'

'No. I'm reasonably sure. But you can never be a hundred per cent sure. Anyway, what's life without a wee bit of risk? Eh? Nae life at all.'

With some misgivings, I accompanied Donnie out of the ward and into the lift. It all went well at first. He didn't seem at all spooked by the presence of so many sinners. He spoke easily as we walked, bought himself a meal of pork casserole and mashed potatoes, and sat and ate with some enjoyment. I sat opposite him. I was beginning to think this wasn't too tricky a gig at all. A slice of gateau, in fact. I looked around and uncoiled a little. If nothing else, I thought, then it's half an hour out of the ward. And not long till home time.

Until Donnie shot bolt upright, capsizing his chair, then hurled his cutlery onto the table with a clash and bellowed, 'I can't eat this!' Spittle flecked his lips. His eyes revolved like Catherine wheels. He was blazing. My heart fell down a lift shaft. From seeming to be a dawdle, this looked like it could now turn into no fun at all. In fact, a complete and utter cast-iron, flame-proof, lifetime-guaranteed fuck-up. Here was I, a quiet and bookish little man, left on his own with the prophet Elijah.

'I can't eat this!'

'Why not?' I asked.

'It's pork! I can't eat pork!'

With anybody else I would have said, 'Well you bought it! Nobody forced you. It was on the menu for all to see, along with the haggis and the fish pie, written in big letters.' But this man was plainly distressed. Instead, I simply said, 'Why not?'

'The Bible forbids it! Aaaargh!'

Actually, it might just have been 'Aargh.' It seemed like a real, four-A, blood-curdling shriek at the time, but that might have been because I was sitting well within the compass of it. Maybe it was no more than a two-A gurgle of agony as he contemplated eternity in the underworld for eating canteen casserole. He was staring at the wall in a fashion not usually associated with sane folk. (I could have wished he'd stared at the menu with as much intensity.) I wondered if he was seeing his equivalent of '*Mene mene . . .*' there. The writing on the wall. Not so much Belshazzar's feast, as poor Donnie's. 'You have been caught eating very ordinary hospital chow featuring lumps of dead pig, and your arse will fry.' Kind of thing. I don't get all that fundamentalist stuff. But Donnie got it in a big way. Maybe Yahweh was still getting through on the internal Batphone. Donnie was a right good conduit of the Lord and all his bad-tempered fussings.

People had stopped eating and were looking at us. Here was a quandary. He was not the kind of man you could tell to sit on his arse and not be so bloody silly. Maybe I should tell him that it was all humbug and to enjoy his casserole. He'd paid £2.40 for it, after all. No. The likelihood was, with the Ancient of Days roaring in his lugs at the time, if I'd tried that one, I'd have been pitched out of a second-floor window as a heretic.

'Didn't you know it was pork when you bought it?'

'No. I'd never have bought pork. Mark 5 . . .'

I thought for a moment he was unhappy with the temperature it had been cooked at.

'Mark 5?'

'Chapter 9. It's the Gadarene swine.'

'Is it? Well, one of them at least, maybe, eh?'

That didn't exactly tickle his ribs. He looked at me scornfully.

'You are a very shallow person, Dennis. Very flippant.'

'I am,' I agreed. 'I confess it is my nature's plague.'

'Not a serious man. There are some things you should be serious about.'

'Well, I can be serious without being solemn. That's the way I look at it.'

'Is nothing sacred to you? There must be something you value.'

I was suitably reproved. He had calmed a little, and I felt sorry for him.

'Don't eat any more, Donnie, if it's making you unhappy.'

He looked at me, worrying.

'You don't think it matters, do you?'

I said nothing. Maybe shrugged a little.

'*Do* you think it matters?'

'If it matters to you, man.'

He softened. After the alarm of his first outburst, here was a good sign. The old Donnie, pre-clozapine, would no more have softened than he would have converted to Buddhism.

'For a sinner, you are not a bad man, Dennis. In there, somewhere, there is a good man.'

'Well . . .'

'I didn't eat of the pig knowingly.'

'Then it's no sin, man.'

He swithered for a few seconds. I could hear the swither slosh about in him. Then he made his mind up.

'I'll have the fish.'

'Leave it to me.'

I took his plate and scraped the Gadarene casserole into the bin. Then I bought him a portion of fish pie. He ate that in contented silence, as if the ingredients included the two fish from the miracle at Bethsaida.

We got back to the ward without any further incident. Charlie told me to write it up in Donnie's notes. And he, Luke and John smirked for the rest of the evening, any time I passed them.

The incident confirmed me as a student of comparative religion, atheist as I am. I took to reading extensively about Islam, Judaism and other world religions. I don't believe any of it. But many people do, and it's important to know what motivates them.

10

There sat down, once, a thing on
Henry's heart
so heavy, if he had a hundred years
& more, & weeping, sleepless, in all them time
Henry could not make good.

John Berryman, 'Dream Song #29'

What motivated Wasim was Islam. He was a young man of twenty-six, of Bangladeshi descent but born in this country. He was handsome: dark-skinned, with liquid brown eyes and a beard trimmed close to his chin. He was also an observant Muslim. In his case his faith was not distorted by his illness or vice versa. There are swivel-eyed fundamentalists in all religions, but Wasim was not one of those. He said his prayers quietly in his room, I believe five times a day, although he was left in privacy to say them. He read the Koran. He ate halal food, prepared for him by the kitchens. And he was quiet, polite and thoughtful. I liked him a great deal. Wasim's problem was that he suffered from periodic bouts of depression.

We got friendly after the time I said to him in Urdu, '_Maaf kijiye, sahib. Khaiiye,_' when I took him his halal meal in his room. He smiled at me and asked, '_Apko Urdu aate hai?_' I had to tell him that, frankly, very little Urdu was coming my way, but I knew how to say, 'Excuse me, sir. Please eat.'

It's a thing of mine – languages. I have always enjoyed learning them, since our class took part in a trial project in primary school French in 1962. I studied French and

Russian at high school, then Italian to O level when I was thirty-eight. Any time we've travelled abroad, I've tried to learn some of the language, at a basic conversational level. I think it's only courtesy to try to speak to your hosts in their own tongue. And it can bring remarkable benefits. I've been misunderstood and taken for a German in France, Italy, Spain and the Netherlands. In Germany I was simply misunderstood. They recognised my Scottish accent for what it was. I learned some of the rudiments of Hindi/Urdu in my previous profession.

And, it was enough to help bond Wasim and me. That and a shared love of cricket. Wasim, like most men with roots in the Indian subcontinent, loved the game and could talk passionately and knowledgeably about it. I am very fond of it too, unlike most Scots, who detest it, regarding it as a symptom of English eccentricity, like morris dancing. But I like it. Clyde, having been born in Jamaica, was obliged by statute to like it. So we sat together and blethered about wood on leather; sometimes all three of us, sometimes just Wasim and me.

Later we moved on to other topics. I said to him that I had always thought that Muslim people were rather wary of being treated in hospital wards where they couldn't be sure of being treated by a fellow Muslim. Or was that just an infidel's ignorance? He said that, by and large, that was the case. On his first presentation here, however, he had been treated by a Muslim psychiatrist who was the senior house officer for the ward at that time. Coincidentally, the current SHO was also a Muslim, by the name of Majeed. Both Wasim and his father had been struck by the kindliness and the good offices of the staff, Muslim or not, and so they had no qualms about his occasional readmittance to the ward.

Anyway, he said to me, was I aware that it was in the Islamic world that the first psychiatric hospitals had been built? No, I said, I wasn't. But every day's a school day. I read up on it. He was right.

Where medieval Christian physicians attributed mental disorder to the influence of the Devil, Islamic physicians of the time proceeded by clinical observation. A more humane attitude is enjoined upon Muslims, in any case, by the Koran. Sura 4:5 (*Al-Nisā*) states, 'Do not give the property with which God has entrusted you to the insane: but feed and clothe them with this property and speak kindly to them.' There's hardly a better recommendation for treatment.

The Persian physician Rhazes wrote two significant studies which recorded clinical cases of his own experience, defined certain illnesses, and described symptoms and treatments. A century later, Avicenna was the first to describe a number of psychiatric conditions such as hallucinations, mania, melancholia and dementia. The medieval Islamic world had indeed pioneered the concept of psychiatric hospitals. The first was built in Baghdad in 705, the second in Fes in the early eighth century, and the third in Cairo in the year 800. Later examples were built in Damascus and Aleppo. Muslim physicians developed several treatments, including psychotherapy, medication, music and relaxation, and occupational therapy. As in many other disciplines, Islamic scholars were ahead of their time.

Wasim's depression was reactive. In other words, its source lay in an external event or events. Reactive depression is a common reaction to intense grief after a bereavement. I believe that Wasim's depression was a profound reaction to the death of his brother in a road accident. His grief was so intense that he had threatened to make an attempt on his own life, in expiation of the groundless guilt he felt at his brother's death. Suicide is expressly forbidden in the Koran. Islam teaches that only God has the right to end an individual's life. His father was extremely concerned, and so he sought expert knowledge to help his son. Slowly and steadily, Wasim had got better. When I knew him, he was on the point of being discharged back into his parents' care. So far as I know, he has never been readmitted.

Wholly different, however, was the case of Wayne.

I reported back to work one Tuesday morning, after a three-day weekend off, to find that Wayne had been admitted from a city hospital. During the morning handover we learned that he was almost completely incapacitated with depression and had been admitted to the ward on a trolley, since he refused to stand or walk; indeed refused to do anything except lie in bed with his eyes shut. He wouldn't eat, wouldn't drink, wouldn't talk. He'd lie in his own shit if nursing staff didn't clean him. Nothing and nobody could jerk him out of his melancholia. His family, his girlfriend, his university pals, nobody. This guy was seriously depressed.

Wayne had what's known as 'endogenous' depression, depression arising from within the patient's mind. It's a psychotic illness. That there was no exterior stimulus for his depression was probable, when I considered that he was young, well-off, clever, successful and had a beautiful girlfriend. If anybody had the right to walk on air and click his heels at every second step, it was him. But life doesn't always work that way.

I took him in a tray of breakfast that first morning. The room door was closed, and the curtains were too. There was a fairly muscular old hum on the air that was obviously emanating from the person of Wayne. I set the tray down on the small chest of drawers at his bedside. Then I opened the curtains and took a look at him.

He lay on his back, with the duvet straight and tight about him. His eyes were closed but I could see them move occasionally under his lids. He was obviously a good-looking young man, if the framed photograph on the table was anything to judge by. It showed him as dark haired and fine featured, in black-tie fig, with his arm around a pretty and curvaceous girl in an evening gown. He was laughing. Now though, as he lay on the bed as rigid as a crusader on a tomb, he presented a sadder sight. He was gaunt. His hair was straggly and collar-length. He had a full set of whiskers. In fact, he looked like a man who has come in from the woods.

'Wayne,' I said, 'I've brought you some breakfast.'

He made no answer. Nor did he move.

'Do you like kedgeree and quail's eggs?'

It wasn't my best joke, and I didn't expect him to guffaw and start slapping his thighs, but he didn't even smile. His eyes flicked under their lids a couple of times as if he was wondering whether to risk opening them to check if those were indeed the ingredients of his breakfast, or whether I was just another barker. Woof woof.

'Well, it makes no difference if you do, because it's only Weetabix and a marmalade roll.'

No reaction. I left. The breakfast tray was still there, untouched, when I returned an hour later.

And, over the next ten days or so, Wayne showed no more animation than that. His parents, well-to-do and concerned for their son, drove from the city every night for visiting time. Sometimes they were joined by his sister. His girlfriend – the one in taffeta in the photo – came out several times too. They sat round his bed like a picture in *Tatler*, held his hand, spoke lovingly to him, urged him to get better, said they would be there for him whenever he needed them, and finally promised to be back the next day. Wayne lay like an effigy.

The man in the street tends to think of depression as just feeling a little down. Having the blues. A dose of the glums. It's not that. It can be a debilitating condition, as Wayne's was. And telling the patient to pull himself together or snap out of it doesn't help. It doesn't do anything, as a matter of fact. It's the psychological equivalent of telling someone with a broken leg to stick a plaster on it and go for a run. A good psychie nurse will know this and never urge a depressive patient to 'cheer up'. What they do, first of all, is ensure that the patient is safe. There are real suicide risks. Then they observe specifically whether the patient is communicating or not, whether there is talk of self-harm or suicide, broken sleep patterns, lowered libido, refusal to eat or inability to attend to personal hygiene. All of these can tell a great deal about a patient.

Wayne ticked the high-risk box on every topic. I'd never seen anything like it. My colleagues who had been in psychie nursing for years had never seen a case as bad. He was non-verbal. He ate nothing. Once in a while he'd suffer a nurse to tip water down his throat. He urinated and defecated where he lay. Two nurses would clean him and change him, rolling him onto his side for the purpose. He made no attempt to resist. He was completely unmoving. Dr Bankstreet consulted Wayne's parents – well, she could hardly consult Wayne. Although she did try, standing by his bed and asking him questions that he never answered.

She prescribed an MAOI – a monoamine oxidase inhibitor, a drug that works by blocking enzymes which stop certain transmitters in the brain. It has an energising effect but is not often prescribed because of the dangerous way it reacts with some foodstuffs. This was, fairly obviously, not a problem with Wayne. But it was impossible to make him take this medication.

Psychiatric patients are notorious for their reluctance to comply with meds. Because of their illness, they often think the medicines are poison. You have to be extremely watchful when giving them tablets – even when they appear to accept them and swallow them before your eyes. They are expert at concealing them under the tongue, or between lip and gum, and then spitting them out when you turn your back. So it was with Wayne. Sometimes he'd refuse to take the pills. Sometimes he'd let the nurse slip them into his mouth and wash them down with water. Or so the nurse thought. Later another nurse would find the pill on the duvet.

Meanwhile, he was not eating and his condition was deteriorating.

11

I sing the body electric.
Walt Whitman

It was obvious that Wayne was not getting better. A blind
man with half an eye could see that. No intervention had
worked. So Dr Bankstreet decided to try ECT. Electroconvulsive therapy – riding the lightning, as we called it in our
less respectful moments. To the layman it seems a barbaric
procedure, still. Hell, it seemed that way to me when we
learned that Dr Bankstreet had prescribed it for Wayne.
Images from movies and memories of anecdotes from the
past combined to make it seem as savage as trepanning.

It's still fairly commonly used for some psychiatric
conditions, especially major depressive ones as experienced
by Wayne. And it's still controversial. There are disagreements over its long-term effects on the patient's brain struc-
ture and general cognition. ('Cognition' is the medical term
for all the ways a person's mind works. Thinking, reasoning,
understanding, memory, the ability to learn new things:
these are all aspects of cognition.)

ECT was developed after psychologists noticed that
depressive patients who also suffered from epilepsy tended
to become lighter in mood after an epileptic seizure. They
wondered if artificially induced shocks might have the same
therapeutic effect. Initial experiments were made with con-
vulsant drugs – including camphor and strychnine – injected

intramuscularly with insulin. And then some bright spark came up with the idea of using electricity.

In 1937 two Italian psychiatrists experimented with ECT on a patient. The story goes that they pondered over just how many volts to zap the poor sod with, and for how long, until they settled on 55 volts for two tenths of a second. The patient was not anaesthetised or sedated prior to being fried. He underwent a major 'grand mal' epileptic convulsion, then sat up, looked around at the doctors and said, 'What the fuck are you arseholes trying to do?' This was a Very Good Thing. Surprisingly. The patient hadn't spoken a word of sense in weeks. Calling his doctors arseholes was a major step forward.

What happens nowadays during ECT is that the patient is given a general anaesthetic and a muscle relaxant. Previously, as described above, there was no anaesthetic. Electrodes are placed on the temples and an electric current is passed across the brain for three or four seconds. The effect is to set off a controlled epileptic seizure. The only visible effect is a slight tremor that runs through the limbs. Compared to earlier times, this tremor is greatly reduced by the muscle relaxant.

The patient wakes later, occasionally suffering from a slight headache or confusion. Or that is the general way of things. But it is not always as straightforward as that. The most common additional side effects are nausea, muscle cramps and cardiac or respiratory problems in patients with tendencies to those conditions. The most distressing adverse effect for many people is short-term memory loss. This occurs most frequently at the time of the ECT course and sometimes for a few weeks after. There may be some loss of past memories too.

While many patients speak positively of the effect that ECT has had upon their illness, it is only fair to balance that with the view of the American novelist Ernest Hemingway. He committed suicide shortly after undergoing a course of ECT in 1961. Before he died he said of the experience, 'What is the sense of ruining my head and erasing my memory, which is my capital, and putting me out of business? It was a brilliant cure but we lost the patient.' Other notable patients who have undergone ECT include the poet Sylvia Plath, singers Lou Reed and Judy Garland, actress Viven Leigh, US TV personality Dick Cavett and an old hero of mine, British blues guitarist Peter Green.

Wayne had five or six blasts of ECT. I was there the first time he was hooked up to Old Sparky, and I watched with fascinated unease as the process unfolded. He had two doses in the first week, with minimal sign of improvement, but after the third dose of Snap, Crackle and Pop the effect was remarkable. He came back to the ward in bed – zonked, as usual. And, as usual, a nurse was delegated to keep an eye on him. I was having a fag at the Nurses' Station when his bedroom door opened and he walked out. Unsteadily, sure. Holding on to the wall for support. Looking like he'd just slept off a weekend bender. But he walked to where I sat with Geraldine and said sleepily, 'Any chance of something to eat? I'm starving.'

Thereafter he progressed rapidly. He ate and drank. He showered. He brushed his teeth. Which was a plus. They had grown so green and furry he probably had to comb them before he could brush them. He shaved and had a haircut. He looked like the guy in the photo again. He was back to his real self.

Unfortunately, his real self turned out to be a spoiled selfish fuckwit, and nobody liked him. But life's like that sometimes.

12

If there be cords, or knives,
Poison, or fire, or suffocating streams,
I'll not endure it.
  William Shakespeare, *Othello*

On admission, the one thing missing from Wayne's presentation had been a suicidal ideation. That apart, he had the full kit. We used to joke that he was too catatonic to bother. That's not true of course. Suicidal thoughts can be present – and acted upon – in the most surprising of cases. One of the commonest reasons for a patient being put on close obs was the risk of suicide. I sat at several doors and bedsides, on the lookout for any attempts at hari-kari. And I've been involved in frustrating actual efforts. Patients tried to strangle themselves with anything that could be used as a ligature: electrical flex, pyjama cords, bras or belts; suffocate themselves with polythene bags; overdose themselves with medicines, and cut their wrists or their throats with knives, razor blades or broken glass. A few tried to drown themselves in the bath. Bathtime was always good for a panic among the staff. The Bathroom was communal and had to be unlocked by one of the nurses. Once inside, the patient could lock the door for privacy, but staff could always open it from the outside in case of emergency.

'You hear any splashing in there?'

'Naw.'

Knock on the Bathroom door.

'You okay in there?'

'Aye.'

'Right. Good. Just checking.'

A pause.

'Gone all quiet in there again, hasn't it?'

'You okay? I said you okay?'

'Best check, Rona.'

A rattle of keys and the door was unlocked.

'Aw, Christ! Dennis, Luke – handers!'

And in we'd have to go and fish them out. Bare backside or not. We reckoned it was better to save their lives than spare their blushes. One guy tried it so often he grew gills. Then it clicked. Maybe he was better having a shower in his room. Or, if he insisted on a bath, somebody had to be in there with him. It was a strange experience to sit on a stool with the crossword while a young man of your slight acquaintance undressed and took a bath. I've rarely wanted to bond that closely with someone.

Patients who are serious about suicide can be very inventive. And resourceful. We once had a patient from London. Albie. He had been found wandering on the motorway near the city. He mumbled something about Loch Lomond when he was admitted but we couldn't make head nor tail of why he was in Scotland. He had no family heritage or ties here. But he was highly motivated towards suicide and we had to observe him extremely closely. Eventually Dr Bankstreet contacted the psychiatric ward he had been attending in London and arranged a transfer. He didn't want to go back, for whatever reason. Maybe he had grown to like the climate here. Anyway. The night before he was due to be returned, a leather necktie was reported missing from the room of another patient with whom he had become friendly. Now Albie was not the formal neckwear type. Strictly smart but casual. So, naturally – as Dickie Valentine didn't sing – the finger of suspicion pointed at him. And, as per the usual procedure, we shut off the bedded area and conducted a search. With special reference to Albie's room.

We found nothing. Charlie was convinced that Albie had snaffled the tie and was hiding it with the intention of using it that night. So he demanded we search the room again. We did. Nothing. No, Charlie insisted, Albie intended to do the Dutch act that night, to escape being returned to London. He was adamant. We went over that room with a fine-tooth cliché. We searched impossible places. We opened up his pillows, guddled about in the cistern in his loo, lifted his lino. We had searched the wardrobe thoroughly – inside and on top. Then Luke suggested we move it. The tie was drawing-pinned to the wall behind it. I've no doubt that Albie would have strangled himself that night in his bed rather than go to London. What horrors, real or imagined, faced him there, I don't know.

Some years ago a friend told me of a visit he'd had from an old girlfriend. She had pitched up at his door one stormy night, shit-faced on drink, saying she couldn't take any more and was going to blow her head off with a shotgun. This girl had never been known to psychiatric services. My friend let her in and noticed that she had a shotgun in the inside pocket of her long waterproof coat. He thought that might not be a positive sign. He fixed her some coffee and listened as she spoke of a series of unhappy events in her life. He provided an ear and a shoulder. Some time later he walked her home and made sure the shotgun was disabled and safe. God alone knows where she'd got it from. But as my pal said, if you are determined to get something these days, you can usually get it. Maybe there's an outlet somewhere called Shotguns R Us. When he regaled me with the story later, over a Singapore sling, he said he had at no time been genuinely concerned. For, said he, he thought, 'Those who talk about it never do it.'

Sorry, but that's bollocks.

This is not the place for a lengthy discussion about suicide risk, but I want to say something about it, for several reasons. The first is that I have been present at several attempts by patients to take their own lives. It is one of the most distressing situations imaginable. It is obviously much more so for the one trying to die, but to be present when another human being makes a serious effort to kill himself or herself, is harrowing in the extreme. Thankfully, no one ever succeeded in Ward 25 when I was there, but a patient did manage to kill herself in Ward 24, the psychiatric ward directly opposite us. I saw the trauma that staff underwent on that occasion. I wish others could be spared that trauma. Second, the effect of suicide on remaining loved ones is overwhelming. Grief, guilt, a sense of stigma, bewilderment, even anger. These are hefty emotions alone. Combined, they can wreck lives. Third, it is important that people acknowledge the scale and seriousness of suicide as a community health problem. Fourth, we need to dispel several myths about suicide, so that future attempts can be prevented.

As many people die from suicide each year as from road traffic accidents. And for each successful suicide, there are at least a hundred more attempts – parasuicides. Approximately 11 to 12 per cent of the population have serious thoughts about suicide at least once in their lives.

Five per cent will attempt it. The old *felo de se* is not an insignificant problem. Some old-fashioned ideas about suicide have to be challenged. Unfortunately, there is a lingering reluctance to discuss the topic. That has to change. It is impossible to know when a knowledge of how to deal with the situation might be needed. And, more to the point, might prove a life-saver. The following points are a summary of current thinking.

Suicide is rarely, if ever, the result of a single traumatic event, such as a death or the ending of a relationship. That single event may provide the spark that ignites the desire for death – the final straw that breaks the camel's back, to change the metaphor – but almost certainly there has been a build-up of events and emotions contributing to suicidal thoughts over time. Time enough to intervene.

Contrary to popular belief, most suicides do not occur with no warning. We can't escape guilt that way. People tell others about how they feel, how they are reacting to certain events in their lives that might be making suicide an option. Their emotional reactions, their behaviour, may indicate their state of mind. And sometimes they just plain tell somebody.

And my pal got it 100 per cent wrong. The notion that folk who talk about suicide never do it is an old one but a wrong one. Just like the flat earth theory. Because people have thought something for a long time doesn't mean it's right. Most people who commit suicide talk about it to somebody first. Such talk has to be taken seriously. Failure to do so might contribute to someone's death. It's as serious as that.

And it's wrong-headed to think that we shouldn't talk about suicide to somebody we think might be at risk.

Serious discussion of suicide does not *increase* the risk of someone committing it; it reduces it. The best way of establishing whether someone is thinking about suicide is to ask them. Talking frankly about suicide and the factors contributing to it are a safety valve, a method of release for the one considering it, and often the thing that prevents it, at least in the short term.

A few other thoughts.

A non-fatal outcome of a suicide attempt does not mean it was mere attention-seeking and therefore not to be taken seriously. Some people dismiss such occurrences as 'simply a cry for help'. *Simply?* If another human being is crying for help, shouldn't we give them all the help we can? A further attempt might not be non-fatal. Most suicidal people are unsure about dying right up to the point of committing suicide. Part of them may want to die, but part of them wants to live. To live better than they have been. Most are looking for a reason not to commit suicide, even if they are unaware of it. And the overwhelming majority of people who are suicidal at some point find a reason to keep living, and a method of doing so. Finally, nor it is true to say that once a person has attempted suicide, they won't again. Previous attempts are a major risk factor.

So. There it is and there you have it. As a wise man once said. I make no apologies to any who feel that the foregoing 700 or so words have been pompous and pious. It is vitally important to be aware of these things. It may save a life. And the life might be yours. Or that of someone you love with all your heart.

And here endeth the lesson.

13

And ne'er did Grecian chisel trace
A Nymph, a Naiad or a Grace
Of finer form or lovelier face . . .
Sir Walter Scott, *The Lady in the Lake*

The ward was unisex. Men and women together, unlike the old asylum, where there were separate locked wards for the sexes. Most of the time this posed no problem. Each patient had his or her own room and most people tended to keep themselves to themselves. But every so often your man Sex would raise his unlovely countenance and cause a problem or two. Well, sex drives most of us mad for at least some of the time. Why should psychiatric patients be any different?

One evening Charlie came up to Clyde, Gordon and me sitting having a fag at the Nurses Station. He informed us that there was a female patient on her way to the ward, transferred from the city. She should arrive within the next half-hour in an ambulance, under escort. She had various problems, which we would learn more about in time, but the main consideration for the moment was that she was sexually disinhibited and would be nursed mainly by female staff. We males would have to be very professional and sensitive in the way we treated her. We nodded sagely and said we understood.

When Charlie went on his way, we were very professional and sensitive. Gordon said that, knowing the ways of the

96

world, sexually disinhibited she might be, but pug-ugly she almost certainly would be. For, he reasoned, where's the problem for a good-looking girl if she likes sex? There would be no shortage of men willing to pamper her, indulge her every whim. Do her the big favour. It followed that this female must have something of the warthog about her. She had the itch, but nobody to scratch it for her. Only reason for that must be she was a misshape with a face that would stop a clock. That's why she'd gone barmy. It all made sense to Gordon. But then Gordon was not Heidegger or Wittgenstein. He didn't spend too much time thinking too deeply. Clyde suggested that maybe the girl's problem wasn't just frustration. Sexual disinhibition, he said, was a different thing. A manifestation of illness. Gordon shut up. But he looked sceptical.

Lesley arrived in the company of two female orderlies from the city hospital. Gordon and I were lingering in the vicinity of the Buffer Zone when she came in.

'Tellt ye,' said Gordon.

The woman who came through the inner door was short and squat – nearly as squat as she was short, in fact. She had lank greasy hair pulled back in a ponytail and held by a rubber band. Her expression suggested that she wasn't the author of that year's *Crack-a-Joke Book*.

'No two pound of her hangin' the right way. Nae wonder the lassie's daft,' whispered Gordon.

'That's one of the escorts,' I said.

'How d'you know?'

'She's got all the paperwork under her arm.'

And so she had. Then Lesley came through the door. She was pretty. Dark brown hair. Bright eyes. Coloured top, blue jeans. She must have been in her mid- to late thirties. She stopped and looked around the vestibule of the ward and at the staff assembled there: me, Gordon, Rona and Pamela. And of course Charlie. She made a wry face. She didn't smile, but she didn't scowl either. She wasn't too impressed. But she certainly wasn't cowed by it all.

Charlie introduced himself, explained the nature of the ward to Lesley, then introduced all of us to her. He concentrated on Pamela and Rona, explaining that they would show her to her room, then orient her to the ward, and be there for her, in case she had any questions or requests on her first night.

'Ey, feyne.' When Lesley spoke, it was in a Belfast brogue so thick you had to strain it through muslin just to make it incomprehensible.

Charlie went into his office with the escorts, to be fully briefed and to take Lesley's notes and files from them. The girls took Lesley up the ward towards the sleeping area. I heard Rona ask her if she was hungry. Lesley said not too, but she could be doing with a sandwich or something.

I looked at Gordon.

'So much for your fucking theory,' I said.

'Christ, I wasn't expecting that. She's a honey.'

'Good-looking woman.' I nodded.

'Fuck, she's a film star,' Gordon said, shaking his head in wonder.

Lesley was shown round the ward. It was almost seven o'clock by then, time for the evening cuppa, so she sat in the dining area and had a mug of coffee and a tuna sandwich. Rona sat with her, to keep her company. Clyde and I rounded up the troops and headed them in the direction of the hatch. They formed a line to the left of the gap and

Ursula served tea, coffee and biscuits. Clyde and I hung around.

Once the cuppas were all doled out, I strolled down the ward to the Smoke Room and blackened a lung. It was Friday evening, not long to home time. A pint or ten. And three days off. I chewed the fat with Luke, Bernard and others. Then I strolled back up the ward to the Nurses' Station. Charlie and Pamela were in the office, writing up notes. Clyde was in there too, hanging around, shooting the breeze, looking cool as a mountain stream and just generally getting in the way. The ward was quiet. Rona sat at the Station, flicking through a magazine. I sat down opposite her.

'New girl in bed?' I asked.

'Aye,' said Rona. 'She's in Room 9. She was just dead beat.'

'Mmm.'

I pulled my paper across the table. There were still a couple of clues in the crossword I hadn't got. I heard John come up. He was at a loose end too.

'Pint the night, wee man?' he said.

I looked up. 'Sure as there's shite in a goat.'

I went back to 12 Across. We heard a room door open and the pad of bare feet. Then Lesley's Belfast twang rang out loudly.

'Whit wan a youse two is gonna make love ta me taneyt?'

I heard a *clunk* behind me. It was John's jaw hitting the floor. I looked up. Lesley stood in the corridor, as naked as the day she was born.

There was nothing nudge-nudge or salacious about the scene, and I don't want to make it sound like there was. The woman was beautiful and in a different context, say an artist's studio, her beauty would have solicited anyone's admiration. But we should not have been seeing her like this. She should not have been naked in a ward corridor, in front of complete strangers. This lassie was severely ill. I guess I dropped out of real time for a second. Rona was the one who jolted the freeze-frame back into life.

'GET INTO THAT ROOM!' she bellowed, and took off from her chair like a ballistic missile. She grabbed Lesley by the shoulders and huckled her round the corner just as a patient called Mike came out of his room. He stopped dead at the sight before him.

'Need any help with that problem?' He smiled.

'JUST KEEP WALKING, MIKE!' Rona yelled.

Mike kept walking. He walked past John and me, who were still staring at each other.

'Now *there's* something you don't often see at supper time,' he said. And kept walking.

Lesley was placed on close obs for the rest of the shift. Rona sat in a chair at her door and would not let her out. (This despite two further attempts by Lesley, now comparatively overdressed in top and pants, to get past.)

When we left that evening there was a female nurse from the night Staff posted at her door.

For several days Lesley continued to present herself in various states of semi-undress, if not complete nudity, and to make extremely coarse suggestions to male staff members. It took a week or two of medication and one-to-one interviews with senior psychiatric staff, all the while under the strict supervision of our female colleagues, before her behaviour started to regularise. The discoveries made about her were typical. Sexual disinhibition may be a symptom of many conditions, but the starting point is often a self-engendered belief that the patient is basically an unworthy individual whom no one would love for herself.

And so it proved with Lesley. She had got in tow with a lowlife boyfriend in the city, a junkie who regularly prostituted her either for drugs, or money to get drugs. He had turned his beautiful girlfriend into a commodity. This kind of depersonalisation is often found at the root of profoundly disinhibited behaviour. The old-fashioned term for the condition, in women, was nymphomania. The corresponding condition in men was once called satyriasis. (I thought that was scaly skin on your elbows, but apparently that's something different.) These terms are no longer considered useful. Clinically, the syndrome is now most commonly described as 'hypersexuality,' and it is recognised as a common symptom of many psychological illnesses.

A few years later we had another disinhibited female admission. This lady was known to the more experienced staff. She had been in the Locked Ward on several previous occasions.

Tilly suffered from bipolar disorder, a condition formerly known as 'manic depression.' Both terms are accurate descriptions of the illness. Sufferers experience troughs of depression but alternate these with highs of manic intensity. When Tilly was manic, she was extremely fond of sex. Not with quite the disinhibition that Lesley showed, but disinhibited enough to indicate to anyone who knew her that she was ill. On this occasion she was admitted wearing a light summer top and a cotton skirt that showed off her newly acquired tan. She was also wearing a straw hat, not on her head but slung around her neck by the chin string, as cowboys sometimes wear their hats in Westerns. And she was carrying a stuffed donkey. Fairly obviously, she had been on holiday when she took ill. And not in Scarborough.

Suspicions had been aroused that she might not be well when she was discovered having sex with a complete stranger in the loo of the plane on the way home from Spain. The crew were alerted to the situation by the uninhibited soundtrack of their activities, as it emanated from behind the locked door. That and the number of irate passengers dancing cross-legged outside it, I suppose. On emergence, she became ratty when admonished by a couple of the cabin crew, and then violent. So she was tied to a seat like a bank manager in a robbery until they landed. Then brought to Ward 25.

She told me later that the sex had been so strenuous that she had burst a blood vessel in her eye. And indeed her left eye was half covered by a bright red film. That's what I call strenuous; almost the dictionary definition of it.

Tilly was a lovely lady, tall and willowy with short blonde hair, and one of the sweetest-natured beings I have ever come across. She knew she was ill, was sometimes upset by the fact, but she faced up to it with extraordinary determination and resolve to get better quickly and get out of hospital. She was kind, loving and giving. Any patient who had run out of smokes went to Tilly. She never refused anyone, always handing over a cigarette – sometimes when she had only a couple herself. If she had sweets, she offered them round before taking one herself.

'You're too generous, Till,' I said to her one time.

'Well, you say that, Dennis,' she said, 'but there'll come a time when I'll need something. And I'll need somebody to help me.'

She was generous with her time and compassion too. Despite the fact that she was ill herself, she would spend ages listening to someone else's woes, giving them her attention, advice and support. Everybody liked her.

For the first few days of that admission she was still worryingly disinhibited. Her help and attention to one of the male patients in his room was a trifle too specialised for Charlie's liking, and earned her a ticking-off. One morning, I was sitting at the Station with Geraldine. I was sucking my pen over the crossword; Geraldine was facing up the bedded area towards Tilly's room. All at once she let out a roar: 'GET BACK IN YOUR ROOM, LADY, AND DON'T COME OUT AGAIN TILL YOU'RE DRESSED!' I almost swallowed the pen. Tilly had been doing a Lady Godiva.

One evening, a quarter of an hour before home time, Charlie and Clyde were shooting some pool in the Games Room. I was dawdling about, watching them and passing smart-arse comments. Clyde was good at the game – he was good at everything he put his hand to – and kept us amused with some banter.

'Rack them suckers up, Chazzeroo. You rack 'em; I'll smack 'em, boah.'

But it wasn't going Clyde's way. Charlie was too good for him that evening. Nothing Charlie tried went wrong; he was playing out of his skin. Now he was lining up a game-winning long pot. He crouched at the top of the table and drew a bead on the black. Tilly was standing with her back to the wall at the foot of the table, smiling and watching.

'Miss it,' Clyde said jocularly. 'This time miss it.'

'I'll make him miss it,' said Tilly, and she lifted her top in one swift movement, from the waist. She was wearing no foundation garment.

'TILLY!' roared Charlie. 'Your room immediately!'

Like a chided child, Tilly stomped out of the room, head down, lip protruding like a wash-hand basin.

'She's no right yet,' muttered Charlie. 'I better go and talk to her.'

And he did. He took Ursula with him to Tilly's room. Charlie was a hugely experienced nurse with a vast reserve of care for the patients in his charge. He talked to Tilly firmly but kindly, explaining that such behaviour was not compatible with her personal dignity – as she knew – and that if she gave the impression by such behaviour that she had no respect for herself, she couldn't really be surprised if others showed her no respect either. Tilly listened like a child and gave her solemn undertaking that it wouldn't happen again. And it didn't. There were no further disinhibited incidents before her discharge a week or so later.

Tilly manages her illness well now. She had a spell in supervised accommodation as a sort of halfway house before setting up a home for herself again, and is doing well. A community psychiatric nurse visits her regularly and administers a depot injection. I've met her on a couple of occasions in town and once on a night out, and she never fails to be pleased to see me, even though I'm somebody she knows from the more difficult times of her life. She is delightful company, with a pawky sense of humour.

'Hello, Dennis! How are you?' she'll yell.

'I'm fine, Tilly. How about yourself?'

'Oh, doin' all right. Managin' to keep my clothes on, at least.'

14

Thou say'st his meat was sauced with thy upbraidings.
Unquiet meals make ill digestions . . .
William Shakespeare, *The Comedy of Errors*

At mealtimes, at least in my first couple of years on the ward, the staff would eat together around one of the dining-room tables, once the patients had all had their meal. Every few minutes we would take it in turn to take a stroll round the ward and check that everything was all right. The sense of bonding and camaraderie that these meals engendered was quite remarkable. I enjoyed them immensely.

Luke was vegetarian, so every day he brought a plastic kitchenware box of something brown and squishy. It didn't matter what the dish actually was – Japanese tofu noodles, butterbean risotto, or chard, sweet potato and peanut stew – it was always an indeterminate shade of brown. Like he'd picked something up from a field and put it in the container. I wasn't sure if all veggie meals looked like that or whether Luke just couldn't cook. He let me try a spoonful of one after I'd commented on its similarity to something shovelled up from the floor of the rhino house. It was delicious. Brown but delicious. He also brought fresh vegetables as a side dish, which at least looked the right colour. And he always had a piece of fruit for his puddin'. He brought a banana one time. Gordon watched him eat his meal, then when he lifted his banana said, 'You gonnae peel that wae your feet?'

Gordon was not a vegetarian. He was a traditional meat-and-two-veg man. Just so long as both vegs were chips. He usually fetched a meal from the cafeteria upstairs and it was always stew or mince and tatties. If it wasn't Scotch pie, beans and chips. His breakfast was often bacon and beans – what Hemingway called 'a pig and the noisy ones'.

Clyde would eat anything. Which surprised me. For a man who was something of an athlete, he packed all sorts of shit into his stomach. Didn't matter what it was – stovies, moussaka, stroganoff, anything – he covered it with a thick coating of Tabasco sauce. Then scoffed it like he hadn't eaten since the old king died. I tried a drop of the sauce once, on the end of my finger. Not a good idea. It was like licking paraffin. I might have used it to clean pennies but I wouldn't have coated my food with it in the way Clyde did.

'You cannae *taste* anythin' under that shit,' observed Gordon. 'It could be sawdust you're eatin' or anythin'. Insects. Old plimsolls. Taste the same with that crap all over them.'

'You mind your own, man,' said Clyde. 'Fuckin' Delia Smith. What you know 'bout cookin'?'

Once Clyde brought in some jerk chicken. He brought in enough to feed a barracks. So I had some. Now that was good! That was the real stuff. Soul food. I've been a fan ever since. But by and large John and I were more traditional in our eating. Charlie always bought something from the canteen. And the ladies usually brought something from home, usually beautifully prepared, which they sat and ate with delicacy and refinement.

The conversation could be startling. Clyde and I might talk about the Test match, until Luke tried to shut us up by remarking that cricket was 'a game for poofs and vicars'.

'Oh yeah, man?' Clyde would say. 'You got Curtly Ambrose bowlin' bouncers at your head at ninety miles an hour, what's that make you? The Pope? Oscar Wilde?'

But Charlie was the one. He always managed to come up with an interesting topic of conversation, one from deep left field that either intrigued everybody or irritated them beyond measure. Mealtimes were a brains trust and culinary experience rolled into one.

'What if,' he said one day at breakfast, 'right? What if your digestive tract was fitted the reverse way from what it is now?'

'What d'you mean?' said John. 'Like, a freak illness?'

'No, no,' said Charlie, 'not an illness or a deformity. I mean, what if everybody's digestive tract was the other way round?'

'Standard issue?' contributed Luke.

'Yep. Everybody's.'

'What if it, then?' I said.

'It would make quite a difference,' said Charlie. 'Just think. Your arse would be where your mouth is . . .'

'Sounds like yours already is,' said Clyde.

'. . . and your mouth would be where your arse is. So, if we were having our meal here, we'd all be naked from the waist down and bent over, facing away from the table, so we could spoon the grub up our mouths.'

'Would revolutionise dinner parties,' I said.

'And if you wanted to kiss somebody goodbye, you'd have to rub arses.'

'Eskimos in reverse,' thought John aloud.

'That would mean,' said Gordon, 'that when you went to the loo, you'd do it out your mouth.'

'No, no. You'd still do it out your arse. It would just be where your mouth is now.'

'So you'd have to wear your pants on your head,' said Rona.

'He does, every Friday night,' said Luke.

'Aye,' said John, 'you havenae thought this through. You'd have to wear your knickers on your head, to hide your arse, and you'd have to breathe through your trousers.'

'Ah,' said Pamela, 'but if your mouth was where your backside is now, then it wouldn't need to be hidden. So you wouldn't need to wear trousers or a skirt down there.'

'Talk about not thinking things through,' I said. 'The flaw in your reasoning is obvious: you make no mention of where one's genitals would be. Would they still be where they are now? In which case, oral sex could possibly take on a whole new dimension. Or would you have your bits up beside your arse, on your head somewhere? Hey? Hah!'

'Which would mean a boom in hat wearing, like in the auld days,' said Luke.

'Never thought of that, did you,' said I. 'And I refute you thus!'

The conversations were generally like that at mealtimes, often covering such diverse issues as how whales mated, when the revolution would take place and – once – why men have nipples. Luke started that one.

'Why do men have nipples?' he wondered over his nut rissole.

'Ah, that's easy,' said Pamela. 'It's all to do with secondary sexual characteristics, isn't it?'

'Yeah,' said Charlie.

'We're all gender neutral at conception,' said Pamela. 'It's during gestation that the foetus becomes male or female. Anyway, both sexes have the same bits, don't they?'

'Do they?' said Gordon. 'I don't think so. I don't have a fanny.'

'You've never had one, have you?' Luke smirked.

'No, you *are* one,' I said.

'Boys!' said Pamela. 'Male and female bits are the equivalent of each other. The clitoris and the penis. The testes and the ovaries. Nipples on breasts.'

'Could I ask you to change the subject, Pamela?' said John, pulling at his collar. 'I'm getting a bit uncomfortable here.'

'Either that, or say it a lot slower.' Gordon smirked.

'What brought this on?' asked Rona.

'The new bloke with the . . . y'know,' said Luke, making a cupping gesture in front of his chest.

'Gynaecomastia?' suggested Pamela coldly.

'That's the one. Him.'

A new male patient suffered from gynaecomastia. It was a common side effect of the antipsychotic drug he was on. This lad had asymmetric gynaecomastia, meaning that one breast was enlarged to womanly size, while the other was not. It didn't seem to upset him in any way, although it did give him an unusual silhouette.

'You know,' I said, 'the really interesting thing about male nipples is not why we have them at all. It's the fact that nipples on men are generally about nine inches apart.'

'Everybody's?' asked Rona.

'Yeah, well, near enough. There will be slight variations in individual cases, I suppose.'

'Mine are much further apart than that,' said Luke.

'Yeah. Well, like I said, there'll be variations.'

'*Much* further. I mean, like, shitloads further.'

'Okay, I'll buy it,' I said. 'How much further?'

'Oh, miles an' miles. I've only got one on me. The other one was removed in Manchester when I was a kid.'

I suspect he started the whole conversation just to build up to that line.

15

The worst of madmen is a saint run mad.
Alexander Pope, *Imitations of Horace*

Sometimes the population of the ward stayed almost static for weeks at a time, with hardly anyone being moved out or in. It depended on the nature of the patients' illnesses. Sometimes progress and improvement were hearteningly quick and a patient could be in and out again in a couple of days. Sometimes the process took weeks, months or even longer.

The commonest method of progressing patients was to move them to the psychiatric ward opposite, Ward 24, when a bed became available. This was a definite upwards move on their personal scale, moving from the Locked Ward to an open one, with consequent improvements in personal freedom. They usually progressed from there to discharge. Occasionally, when Dr Bankstreet thought it appropriate, a patient was discharged straight from 25 into their parents' or spouse's care.

At the time of which I speak there had hardly been any movement for over two weeks. Then, as is commonly the case, there was a flurry of activity. Bernard and Harriet went. Archie went. And Donnie got sufficiently better to be moved back to his original presenting hospital.

'Somewhere near Aberdeen?' I asked.

'Either that or somewhere near Corinth,' Luke thought.

'Corinth?' wondered Gordon. 'Why Corinth?'

'The Bible. The First Epistle of the Apostle Paul to the Corinthians.'

'Eh?'

'It was a joke.'

'Not a very funny one.'

'Not now,' I agreed. 'Now that we've anatomised it. What is it they say? You can dissect humour like you can dissect a frog, but it always dies when you do it. Once you've pulled the wings off a joke to see what made it fly, it can't fly any more.'

'Who said that?'

'Me.'

That Donnie was able to be discharged at all was due to the antipsychotic drug clozapine. It is normally used only as a last resort, in cases of schizophrenia that have proved resistant to any other form of treatment. And the reason for this is that it can cause a serious condition called agranulocytosis. This condition involves a severe lowering of the white blood-cell count. It has led to death in some patients, from a severe lack of one kind of infection-fighting cells. The body's immune system is suppressed, and as a result sufferers are at dangerously high risk of serious infections.

But the drug is more arguably effective than anything else for treating schizophrenia, and can also prove extremely beneficial in reducing suicide risk in that illness. So patients prescribed clozapine need to have frequent blood tests to monitor their white cell count. Initially, patients are monitored weekly. Results were given to patients in Ward 25 using the traffic lights analogy. Green meant no problems. Amber meant there was a situation worth watching. Red meant that there was evidence of a lowered white cell count and the patient had to come off the drug.

If there were no reds in the first six months, then the patient could be moved on to two-weekly monitoring, and then four-weekly, so long as results merited it.

It worked well enough for Donnie, and so four beds were empty when I left the ward that Friday for the big weekend off. But beds seldom remained empty in the IPCU for long. There was a corresponding whirl of admissions, and by the time our shift arrived for a new week on the following Tuesday they were occupied again.

Donnie had just gone – in fact, the doors had just closed on his evangelical coat tails – when Stanislaus was admitted. He too had a dose of that Ole Time Religion. (The religious nut jobs of the world are a constant quantity.) But, unlike Donnie, Stanislaus was a Catholic. He was what Luke called a 'spoiled' priest, having studied for the priesthood for two years in a seminary in his native Ireland. He had a missal that he consulted at regular hours of the day. He got a visitor to bring in his statuette of the Virgin Mary, and he placed it reverently on his windowsill between two little jars of flowers. And he was often to be found on his knees at prayer before it when a staff member entered his room to advise·him of meals or visitors.

He was a good-looking man, maybe in his mid-fifties, born in County Clare, with a soft and mellifluous Irish accent. By no means an idiot, he could converse knowledgeably about many topics, artistic and scientific. And he had of course studied fairly esoteric subjects in the seminary like Hebrew and dogma. We were never sure quite why he had discontinued his studies and he showed a marked disinclination to tell us. He was equally unforthcoming about how or why he had come over the water and settled in Scotland.

Possibly because of his training, he almost always brought any subject back to religion, or gave the Catholic slant on whatever we were talking about. It got remarkably tedious, remarkably quickly. And this was the key to his problem. He could not keep from loudly and pointedly reminding non-Catholics how secondary they were in the eyes of God, and how they would surely suffer the agonies of the damned, if they did not convert to Rome pronto.

He lived alone in a flat in a poor area of a town that was notorious for being a hotbed of anti-Catholic feeling. Quite how justified this rep was, I'm not sure – at least as regards the whole town. It seems though that the particular street in which Stanislaus lived housed several members of the local Orange Order, or so he claimed. He also declared that every second house in the street was the home of a Rangers supporter. Or a family of them.

We were talking in one of the Interview Rooms one day.

'Do you have problems with the neighbours, Stanislaus?'

'Call me Stannie. Everybody calls me Stannie.'

'Sure. You have neighbour problems, Stannie?'

'They complain when I play my music, Dennis. And I have every right to play my music.'

'Yeah? What do you play? The Stones? Led Zep?'

'Father Sydney MacEwan.' And then he started to sing: 'O Mary, we crown thee with blossoms today, Queen of the Angels and Queen of the May.'

'Cannae see why anybody would take exception to that,' I said, smiling.

'It's a beautiful hymn to Our Lady, Dennis,' replied Stanislaus in a slightly huffy voice.

'Sure. Maybe not the most tactful thing to play in your street, though, Stannie, eh? At least, not loudly. Were you playing it loudly?'

'Not at first, Dennis. At least, I didn't think it was loud. But when they started kicking my door and bumping on the floor from underneath with a brush, I just thought, to hell with you, you Orange bastards, and I turned it up full vol.'

'What did they do then?'

'They kept kicking my door. And they yelled through my letter box.'

'Oh yeah? What'd they yell – *Dominus tecum*? "Faith of Our Fathers"?'

'They called me a Fenian bastard.'

'Mmm. See any irony in that?'

He didn't, of course. Holy Joes don't do irony, as a rule. Holy Joes of any shade or stripe. They're never comfortable with nuances, with subtle distinctions. They much prefer monochrome. They see the world in black and white. Good people go to church (the correct one of course), believe all the dogma they're fed without questioning any of it and, as a consequence, end up sitting on a cloud in a Wee Willie Winkie nightgown, strumming a lyre on the right hand of the Father. Bad people are everybody else, basically. Especially people who go to different churches or read different holy books. And they get the Burning Fire with wee imps jabbing their backsides with tridents. It's a simplistic viewpoint. Black and white. Living on a chessboard.

Now, had that been me in that situation, living as a Catholic surrounded by fairly eager members of the Orange Order and supporters of Rangers FC, I'd have kept my head down. I'd have done the same if I'd been a Rangers supporter and a staunch Protestant in an enclave of Catholic

Celtic men. For the simple reason that I'm rather fond of my head and I'd like to keep it attached to my neck. I certainly would not have played Sydney MacEwan singing hymns to the Virgin Mary at the volume of a full-throated roar. It's a survival thing. I think most of us would be the same.

Not Stannie.

He went out sporting the green and white hoops of Celtic and wearing a rosary as a neck chain. He continued to play Catholic sacred music loudly and ignore the catcalls. He fashioned a little shrine to Our Lady on his windowsill, just to advertise his devotion to anyone who cared to look up three floors and see it. I doubt many did. At least no one had thrown stones at it. He did tell me that he was shoved around one evening on his way home from Benediction. Some louts were hanging about and jostled him a bit, calling him a misbeliever and a cut-throat dog and spitting on his Catholic gaberdine.

'They threatened to kick seven different colours of shite out of me, Dennis.'

'Well, seven is a mystical number, Stannie. Think about it. The Seven Gifts of the Holy Ghost. Seven hills of Rome. Jinky Johnstone was number 7. Seven little girls sittin' in the back seat, kissin' and a-huggin' with Fred . . .'

He did laugh; I'll give him that. But he was annoyed at my flippancy.

'I'm being serious, Dennis,' he protested. 'They threatened me with grievous bodily harm.'

'Well, if I was you, I'd keep a low profile for a while. You can still be as devout and devoted to your religion without ramming it up other people's noses.'

'That's what the police said.'

'Oh? You went to the police?'

'Yes, and they said what you said. Don't shove it down other people's throats.'

'No, I said don't ram it up their noses.'

'Yes, well, they're ramming their beliefs up my nose. Why are they right and I'm wrong?'

'There's more of them.'

'Is that what you have instead of principles?'

'No, that is a governing principle of mine. To keep myself in one piece.'

Stannie was disgusted. If he'd been familiar with the word 'pusillanimous', he might have called me it. He wore his faith like a badge. More, like a burning brand. He strutted about in a state of grace. He took his meal from the hatch, found a place and, no matter who he was seated beside, joined his hands, made the sign of the cross, bowed over his plate and said grace loudly. Not everybody appreciated it.

'Bless, us, O Lord, and these thy gifts—'

'What ye daein'?' said Alfred one lunchtime, pausing in his repast to look at the praying Stannie.

Stannie finished grace and blessed himself again before he looked briefly at Alfred, picked up his cutlery, shifted his gaze to his meal and answered curtly as he took a forkful, 'Saying grace.'

'Well, dinnae.'

'Why not? Are you a Protestant? This is a dark Protestant land, right enough.'

'Naw, I'm nuthin'. But I don't like aw that mumbo-jumbo stuff.'

'Mumbo-jumbo? No, that's the teaching of our Holy Mother, the Church. And I'm perfectly entitled to practise my faith without interference.'

'Well, away an' practise it somewhere else, then.'

'I can say my prayers wherever and whenever I choose, without interference.'

'If I was interferin', you'd ken aboot it,' growled Alfred, and went back to his fishcakes.

I was standing in the Dayroom one afternoon, looking wistfully out of the window and wishing things were other, when Stannie materialised at my side.

'Dennis,' he said, 'do you believe in God?'

'Which god?' I said.

There was an appalled intake of breath. I might as well have suggested that we sack the Convent of the Little Flower, topple all the images, pillage the plate and finish by converting the nuns to Mormonism. He looked at me like I was the seed of Belial whose name was Zabulon.

'There is only one God; God the Father Almighty, creator of heaven and earth.'

'You say. What about Jove? Zeus? Thor?'

'Pagan gods.'

'But gods nonetheless. And each one, in their day, worshipped with exactly the same fervour that you worship yours. No, I don't believe in God, Stannie.'

His eyes filled and he looked at me with benevolent and saintly compassion, the yearning of a good shepherd for a sheep that is lost. It was the most nauseating expression I've ever seen on anyone.

'I'll pray for you, Dennis,' he said. 'I'll pray that you may come back to the Lord. In fact, I'll pray for you now. Pray with me! Pray with me now. You shall be saved.'

He sank to his knees and joined his hands.

'Stop it,' I said with an embarrassed giggle. 'People are lookin'.'

It was true. People in the armchairs by the television were watching our little Miracle Play with some interest.

'Our Father, who art in heaven . . .'

'Get up, Stannie! This is the sort of thing you should do in the privacy of your own bedroom.'

'. . . give us this day our daily bread . . .'

As I'd found out with Donnie, you can't get through to fundamentalists. I made an excuse and left.

16

What are you mad?
I charge you, get you home.
William Shakespeare, *Othello*

The aforementioned Alfred was a giant of a man, built like a linebacker and with a hair-trigger temper on him when he was unwell. I don't think Stannie realised just how near to martyrdom he had been that time. Like so many patients, Alfred was entirely the opposite when he was well. Then he was a shy man, quiet and unassuming. If he was ill enough to be in hospital, though, extreme care had to be taken around him.

This was the only admission he had in the seven and a half years I worked in the Locked Ward, although he had been in the asylum on many occasions. One of the best things about working in a ward like 25 was that, unlike in Care of the Elderly, you saw people getting better and moving on. Sometimes the process was extremely slow and intermittent, granted. But it took place eventually. The downside of this was that some patients, having spent time on the ward and benefited from the regular programme of medication, got out and, because they felt better, assumed that they were completely cured. So they stopped taking their meds. Didn't need it. Felt great. And they got ill again. Pretty soon they were back in the IPCU, going through the whole rigmarole again. The revolving door syndrome.

Alfred had been like that. In and out like a fiddler's elbow. I watched him walk up the ward the day he was admitted. Big. Strong. Glowering. He held his head erect and looked contemptuously from side to side at us lesser mortals. It was the sort of entrance that a heavyweight boxer makes through the audience before climbing into the ring.

'He looks like he'd be handy,' I said to Luke.

Luke nodded. 'Takes about six of us to restrain him when he goes off it.'

My heart soared like a lark at this intelligence.

In point of fact, it was not to be long before I was involved in my first restraint, but it was not with Alfred. Because he had been in before, the guys knew him and counselled me to take great care around him. Alfred complied with the medication Dr Bankstreet prescribed for him, but he was extremely anxious to get out of 25 and back to the outside world. So much so that he constantly harped on about it, to every member of staff he met, at every opportunity that presented itself.

'Nurse, when dae ah get oot ae here?'

'Oh, that's up to the doctors, Alf.'

'You aw say that.'

'That's because it's the truth.'

'But ah'm better. Ah should be at hame.'

'You are better, Alf. And I'm sure it won't be long till you are home.'

He'd shake his head, growl like a bear and lumber off. Sometimes he'd favour you with a fierce glare before going. It didn't suggest sweetness and light were uppermost in his mind at that point. And if he met another staff member two paces up the corridor, he'd go through the same dialogue. 'Nurse, when dae ah get oot ae here?'

Things came to a head. Like a boil.

Dr Bankstreet was an extremely able and experienced consultant, but she was also an extremely busy one. Accordingly (now, there's a delightfully quaint adverb to start a sentence with), her services were augmented by those of a senior house officer, a junior colleague who could be on the ward for at least some time, every day of the week. And could be bleeped whenever necessary. For example, to interview a new admission. SHOs worked on the ward for six months and then moved on, to be replaced by another. The SHO conveyor belt delivered some interesting characters to us over the years.

At the time of Alfred's last admission the SHO was a psychiatrist called Humphrey. Humphrey was a rotund and jovial fellow, smiling and witty, who always dressed in a dark three-piece suit with a watch and chain. He cracked jokes, took a pint, supported Liverpool and was scathing about Scottish football. He had an eye for the ladies. And he swore like a trooper with the boys. Usually about Scottish football. He was a latter-day version of Falstaff. He was a genuine Scouser and, although he had adopted an RP (i.e. posh) accent, was perfectly capable of stripping the features off someone who had annoyed him with a blast of pure Knowsley.

'Well, Humph,' I would say, 'I see Man U humped you guys at the weekend.'

'Manc bastards.'

'Ho, we're talking class football here. No like that shite you support.'

'Ah! you can get yourself to fuck! Shite! You talk to me of shite! What about Celtic? Hey? Rangers? My friend, Scottish football is shite! And my name isn't Humph. It's Hum-*free*. Mind it.'

Gordon walked by once when we were sprinkling each other with witticisms in this way. He stopped, listened and then smirked at Humphrey.

'Aw right dere?' he said in an appallingly bad Scouse accent. 'But dey doo do, don't dey?'

Humphrey looked at him. Then he looked at me and John.

'Worra prickh!'

Anyway. Humphrey promised Alfred one evening that he would see him the next day. Alfred had latched on to him, like a terrier to a trouser leg, the moment he'd set foot on the ward.

'When am ah gettin' home, Doc? Eh? Ah feel great. When am ah gettin' home?'

'I will see you tomorrow, Alfred. Tomorrow, all right? Ver-ry busy today. Very busy.'

'Ah want tae go hame.'

'Yes. Tomorrow. I will talk to you tomorrow.'

And Humphrey slipped into the relative sanctuary of the office to make a phone call and complete the one or two pressing tasks he had on hand. Alfred strolled off. In his mind Dr Humphrey had told him that he would be going home the next day. The word tomorrow had been uttered. And everybody knows what 'tomorrow' means. Alfred certainly knew. If only he had considered the words of the immortal John Lennon. For assuredly tomorrow *never* knows.

Alfred was a ray of sunshine for the rest of the evening. A great big six-foot-one twenty-stone ray of sunshine. He beamed so broadly that even Evan, who noticed very little about anybody else, commented on it as they queued for the evening cuppa.

'Looking happy.'

'Aye. Gaun hame tomorrow. Doctor tellt me.'

Stannie, one place before Alfred in the queue, turned round and smiled at him.

'That's great news, Alfred. I'm pleased for you.'

'Thanks. You're no gonnae say a prayer aboot it, are you?'

Stannie smiled tolerantly.

'Not here. But I will thank God for your sake when I say my prayers tonight.'

Alfred approached the hatch and accepted a cup of coffee and a stack of digestive biscuits from Luke. Luke looked at Alfred's grinning dish.

'Full of the joys tonight, Alfie?'

'Gaun hame the morra, Luke. Dr Humphrey tellt me.'

Clyde approached him when he moved away from the hatch. 'Actually, Alfred, I don't think that's what Dr Humphrey said. He said he would *see* you tomorrow. You know, talk about it tomorrow? When he has time?'

Alfred stopped and glared at Clyde.

'He said tomorrow. I said I wanted to go hame. And he said "*tomorrow*",' Alfred explained with great precision and patience.

'All I'm sayin', man, yeah,' said Clyde, 'is don't build your hopes up too much. Okay? You might have misinterpreted what he said. I don't want to see you disappointed. Nobody does. Alf – yeah?'

Alfred stood, coffee and biscuits in hand, brows lowered, and brooded for a second or two.

'Ah better *no* be disappointed the morra,' he said. Then he strode over and sat before the TV to enjoy his snack.

Clyde strolled over and joined me where I stood at the hatch. Luke leaned on the sill of the hatch and looked out.

'Whhh!' said Clyde. 'I sure as hell hope Humphrey gonna let him home tomorrow. Alfred gonna spit his dummy out if he don't.'

'Nae chance,' said Luke. 'The big man's no right for it yet. He's better, but he's no right. He'll have to get time out first, for one thing.'

I must have looked unhappy. I felt it.

'Are we gonnae be fightin' the morra?' I asked.

'Looks like it,' said Luke.

'Hope Humphrey can ride a punch,' said Clyde as he wandered away.

Next day I was actually at the top end of the ward when it happened. Thankfully. Rona and I were impersonating maids in a Dutch genre painting at the time. I was handing her laundered bedlinen, still slightly warm, from a huge metal trolley and she was folding it neatly before she put it away, equally neatly, in the linen cupboard.

From the bottom of the ward, we heard raised voices – no, we heard *a* raised voice – and then a slammed door, quickly followed by an almighty thump and a yell of agony. Rona hissed, 'God! What's happened?' Then the alarm started its electronic *mee-maw*. And I, much against my better judgement, took off down the ward to where the shindy was coming from.

I was not unhappy to see that John and Charlie were already frogmarching Alfred up the ward, with Luke and Clyde in attendance behind, like Ladies of the Privy Chamber. Alfred was not struggling; he was meekly allowing Charlie and John to take his arms and march him. He kept saying, 'Ah'm okay, boys. Honest. Ah'm okay.' But his right hand was inflating like a balloon even as he walked.

I grabbed Luke as they drew level.

'Did he wallop Hum-*free*?'

'Naw,' hissed Luke, his eyes expressing the profoundest admiration, 'he punched the windae out the Smoke Room door.'

And then he walked on. Naturally, I went down to the Smoke Room. Pamela and Gordon were chivvying a scatter of patients away from the area. There was a drift of glass snow on the tiles of the Smoke Room floor. It had once been the toughened glass square in the door.

'My God!'

Pamela made eyes and nodded. Yeah, she thought so too. There was no sign of Humphrey in the office when I went in quest of him. I was still there when Luke came back down the ward.

'Hum-*free* do a runner?'

'Out that door like shite out a goat,' confirmed Luke. 'Just as soon as Alfie punched the window out.'

'Smart move.'

'Slick fuckers, these SHOs,' said Luke. 'For a fat Scouser, he didnae half haul ass.'

'Alf getting his backside perforated?'

'Nah. Took two and five okay.' (A does of meds.) 'He's just gettin' his hand bandaged. Prob'ly broke every fuckin' bone in it.'

Later I was having a drag when Alfred came into the Smoke Room. His hand was encased in bandages. He smiled sheepishly and sat down.

'Sore paw?' I said to him.

'Aye. That was stupid.'

'Because Dr Humphrey wouldnae let you home?'

'Because he wouldnae speak to me. Said he would get back to me. He had things to dae first.'

'These guys are busy, Alf. He'd a got round to you eventually.'

'Yeah. But he sayed he would let me hame the day.'

'Naw. Clyde told you you'd picked him up wrong. He meant he'd *see* you today.'

'But he didnae see me. He kept puttin' me aff.'

'Pretty violent thing to do,' I said, nodding at the door, where two very quiet workmen were even then replacing the glass.

'Well,' he said, 'it was either that or Dr Humphrey. An' I thought it was better that I hurt the glass than a doctor.'

That gave me pause. In the midst of his towering rage the big fella had thought better of giving Humphrey a tanking and had lamped the door instead. I found that really impressive. It was just as well for Dr Humphrey, too. That punch might well have severed his head from his body. He'd have had to pick it up and do his entire ward round carrying it under his arm, like the Green Knight.

The next morning Charlie took Alfred out for a stroll round the grounds. It went well. In the afternoon Charlie came upon Luke, John and myself having a gasper at the Nurses' Station.

'Dennis,' he said, 'Alfie's got another half-hour time out. He wants to go to the garage for fags. Will you take him? I need Luke and John here for an admission.'

'Sure,' I piped.

This was a common time out. Many, if not most, of the patients smoked. When they got the opportunity, they liked to walk to the filling station near the hospital and buy their supply of wheeze. The hospital shop, strangely enough, did not stock fags. When patients were not allowed out, they often asked staff to fetch them. Glumly I ground my own stub in the ashtray and stood up.

'Oh well,' I said. 'I'll check if anybody else wants anything.'

'You be careful the big man disnae throw you onto that garage roof,' chortled John.

'Aye.' Luke laughed. 'He could land you up there with one of his punches.'

'Mind,' urged John, 'if he runs away, dinnae chase after him.'

(This was actually ward protocol. If a patient on escort ran off, staff were advised not to pursue. The man in the street would not see an affronted nurse chasing an absconding psychie patient; he would simply see one man chasing another – sometimes a big fit man chasing a slighter character. Chances are, if he intervened, it would be to come to the patient's assistance, not the nurse's.)

'Fear not my government,' I said.

Luke laughed again. 'But run like hell if he starts chasing you.'

'If he chased me, he'd *never* catch me,' I said emphatically.

'How no?' said John. 'You don't look that athletic to me.'

'I'm not,' I said. 'But it wouldn't matter. Because he'd be slippin' in my shit all the way along the road.'

17

And Something's odd — within —
That person that I was —
And this One — do not feel the same —
Could it be Madness — this?

Emily Dickinson, 'Poem: 410'

And then there was the first restraint I took part in.

Evan was a patient on the ward when I joined the staff and had been for some time. A fifty-year-old Welshman, his diagnosis was Asperger's syndrome, but Dr Bankstreet suspected that he had an underlying psychosis as well. It took a long time for the psychosis to manifest itself, but she was right.

Asperger's is a condition that is closely related to autism. Indeed, some psychiatrists think that it shouldn't be thought of as separate, as it is really only a high-functioning version of it. Like autism, Asperger's is characterised by a lack of social skills, awkwardness in personal relationships, and restricted and repetitive interests. Unlike full-blown autism, there is no obvious lack of cognitive or language development.

Evan, typically, found it difficult to relate to and interact with people. He had no friends. Conversation with staff was stilted. He either uttered monosyllables or, rarely, engaged in long-winded and rambling stories about pet obsessions. Coal mining was one; cage birds another. These showed little sign of stopping and needed no input from the listener. He had poor eye contact and little facial expression.

As with many sufferers from the condition, Evan was physically clumsy and awkward in his gait. But he was immensely strong. This, allied to his difficulty in interpreting any communication other than on the most strictly literal level, could cause serious problems. Evan was perfectly capable of misunderstanding Humphrey's remark, as Alfred had done. Indeed, judging from their presentations, he was the more likely to do so. Once or twice on the ward there had been episodes. Evan would be observed to be smouldering for a few days – nobody could establish why – and then he'd explode. Most days Evan sat wrapped up in himself by the TV with his litre bottle of Coke. In the afternoons he would go to his room and draw or listen to his music. Sometimes he took part in activities in the GP Room, where he did the same things or played computer games. He was generally happiest in his own company.

And so, most days, there was no problem. Not this day.

It was lunchtime. Evan had been muttering and stomping about with a black look on his face for most of the morning. Pamela had sat by him and tried to involve him in conversation, but he was having none of it. She looked significantly at John and me as she stood up and turned from him. I knew what that look meant. Loins would have to be girt. I just knew that this was my time. Shortly I would be involved in a physical restraint. Evan might have been ungainly in physical terms, but he was as strong as Stinking Bishop. This would be the one. There was no chance of me being broken in on a weedy librarian with an obsessive-compulsive disorder.

I was standing by the big windows as the patients finished their lunches. Evan returned his tray to the hatch and strode off to his room, to return with a new litre bottle of cola.

'Aw right, Evan?' I asked, nodding at him and then returning to a conversation I'd been having with one of the female patients.

I could sense he was behind me and my skin crawled. I flinched just as he raised the bottle to wallop me over the head with it. John had been at the hatch and saw it. Luke just at that moment entered from the corridor and saw it too.

'Evan!' he yelled.

Both John and Luke were there in seconds and pinioned his arms.

'You aw right, wee man?' said John.

'Aye. Just felt he was going to give me one on the crust with the bottle there.'

'He was. Pam!'

Pamela came in, saw the situation and nodded. She headed off to the Treatment Room for some medication. They released Evan.

'Stay here,' said John.

'I did nothing,' Evan mumped. But he stayed.

Pamela came back with the regulation two and five, and a cup of water to wash them down.

'Take these, Evan.'

'What are they?'

'To calm you down.'

'No!' he yelled and smacked the pills out of Pamela's proffering hand. Then made to swipe her.

On the instant, John and Luke had him and wrestled him abruptly to the floor. The C & R training kicked in and I had Evan by the legs the minute he hit the ground. We turned him onto his stomach, John and Luke mirroring each other at Evan's shoulders, restraining his arms. I held his legs beneath the knee, tight into my side to minimise bruising as he struggled. And boy, did he struggle! He bucked like a bronco. He flipped his back like a salmon. He wanted to kick the shit out of us. Understandably. He was angry and resentful. And probably more than a little frightened himself. But the restraint was tested and tried. He was as stuck as an Elastoplast and tired pretty quickly.

I'm glad he did. In all my time on the ward the one thing I hated was being involved in restraints. I'm not the strongest man in the world and I've never been a fighter, so I derived no pleasure from it. More importantly, I was always conscious of *their* fear and hurt, and the pain that they might be going through. Not physical pain – hopefully – because the holds were designed to avoid that, but the mental pain it could cause. The indignity. The affront to an often fragile sense of personal identity. I think everyone felt the same. Sadly, there were times when physical restraint was unavoidable.

Pamela, having exited the scene to prepare an intramuscular injection, returned and applied it. She tugged his jeans and pants down till the upper quadrant of his buttock was visible, then jabbed him. After five minutes Evan was lying calmly.

'You okay now?' said Luke. 'Evan, you going to behave if we let you up?'

'Yes.'

'Right. Dennis is going to let go your legs. If there's any trouble, we'll apply the restraint again. Understood?'

'Yes.'

I released his legs and stood up. Slowly John and Luke let go of his upper body and we stepped away from his prone figure. After a moment he pushed himself to his feet and wandered away to his seat by the TV. I don't know why he took a breenge at me that day. Unpredictability – what terrifies many people about mental illness. But he did similar things at random times to different people.

* * *

After waiting some time to be involved in my first restraint, I was involved in several more in quick succession thereafter.

There was a young lad who was transferred from a hospital to the north of our catchment area. He didn't stay long with us. In fact, he got a lot better quickly. But while he was with us he took exception to Clyde. Clyde had got used to cheap insults from racist bigots over the years – indeed, he took that neanderthal guff in his stride – but this guy, rather than start with catcalling, racial insults or offensive gestures, went straight to violence. When Clyde stood before him that first morning they met, with his meds in a cup and a drink of water, the young man did precisely what Evan had done. He smashed the drugs out of Clyde's hand. Then he swung a punch at him. Luke and I happened to be steps away when Clyde set off his alarm.

We rushed in. Clyde was holding him off as he swung punches. Luke took an arm; Clyde did the same, and I secured his legs. Same as before. But one of the things about the lad was that he wasn't too fussy about his toilet. I don't mean he would do it anywhere. Not that. He did it in the right place. He just wasn't too particular about personal hygiene or changing his underwear. We may be talking abstersion of the podex here. Or lack of it. Poorly absterged or otherwise, I was too near that podex for comfort. It was not fragrant. Floribunda it was not.

When we let him up I told the guys about it.

'How about somebody else taking the business end next time?'

Clyde smiled. 'You doin' just fine.'

And, despite my protestations and complaints that dealing with the lower half of the body wasn't the best position, most restraints where I was involved in future were carried out the same way. Dennis was the bum guy.

18

More matter for a May morning.
William Shakespeare, *Twelfth Night*

Another weekend in the wide world and two more new admissions when we returned.

Voytek was a young Pole. Tall, thin-featured and haughty as the Earl of Hell, he barely spoke. When he did deign to address us or answer a question, his English was excellent and delivered in an incongruously soft accent. His hair was shaved closely into the wood; he wore narrow wire eyeglasses and had a vaguely scholarly look. He might have been a crazed wizard. Or a scientist who had discovered evolution the day before Darwin published *On the Origin of Species*.

Most of the time he dressed in desert camouflage army fatigues, including the cap. He wore a German Iron Cross on a string round his neck. His footwear was invariable – army issue, black leather, high-leg combat boots. He cut quite a figure on the way to the Smoke Room, striding along the ward like Stormin' Norman. But this was by no means his entire military wardrobe. When winter came, and the wind howled around the courtyard, Voytek put on an air force greatcoat and went out for half an hour, circling the yard like a solitary prisoner in the compound of some Stalag near the Russian Front. On high days and holidays or, as Gordon put it, when he was 'supremely bonkers', he would tog up in the fatigues, the boots and the greatcoat, and top it all off with a leather flying helmet complete with ear flaps, chinstrap and goggles. I found the choice of clothes strange. Disdainful he might be, but he was in no way an aggressive man, nor did he appear to be especially interested in military matters.

He suffered from bipolar disorder, but his diagnosis and treatment were complicated by the fact that he also had epilepsy. As if to prove the theory behind ECT – that patients get brighter after an epileptic seizure – immediately after Voytek had one, he became quite cheery. Well, cheery for Voytek. He might even initiate conversations himself, something he never did otherwise.

Epilepsy is an extremely complicated condition, although an epilepsy website defines it simply as 'a tendency to have recurrent seizures (sometimes called fits)'. These fits happen when an unexpected surge of electrical activity interrupts the way nerve cells pass signals to each other in the brain. There are many different types of seizure but the kind Voytek suffered from are known as 'tonic clonic' seizures. This jingling title refers to the kind of muscle spasms and contractions that characterise them. Most people would call them convulsions.

Voytek would suddenly stiffen, in the midst of any activity, say, playing pool, and then fall. On the floor he would jerk and shake convulsively, and his breathing would become harsh and croaking. The first time I saw it happen, it was most alarming. He was tall and thin, like I say. Striding along the corridor, he suddenly stopped, stiffened and fell like a roll of linoleum. My first instinct was to rush to his assistance, but Clyde advised me not to; to stand back. My safety was important too, he said. So long as there was nothing in Voytek's immediate vicinity that could harm him if he hit it, I should leave the seizure to run its course. When he was coming out of it, Clyde said, he was unaware of his surroundings or what was happening to him, and he had been known to lash out.

'Don't hold him down,' Clyde said. 'And don't stick nothin' between his teeth, like you see in the movies. He can't swallow his tongue just now, no matter how much it look like he could.'

'How do you know so much about this?'

'My old man was epileptic. It's pretty common.'

The real fear with Voytek was that he wouldn't come out of the seizure but would continue to have recurrent fits – what is known as 'status epilepticus', or just 'status'. That's a medical emergency. It happened once or twice, usually when Voytek was not complying with his medication. I have said before how tricky it can be to ensure that some patients are taking the medicines they need. This is especially so when patients who have ordinarily been no problem take it into their heads to stop, for whatever reason. They might be seen to put the pill in their mouth and go through all the actions of swallowing, as they have always done. Meanwhile the pill is under the tongue or secreted elsewhere in the mouth. Then, when they're alone, down the john it goes. Staff vigilance is essential.

When Voytek went into status, trained staff had to administer a diazepam suppository. diazepam acts quickly and its effects are long-lasting. Meanwhile, another staff member would be bleeping the duty doc. Status epilepticus emergency. It was that dangerous.

But it was amazing just how bright Voytek got after a seizure. It didn't last a whole long time, but it was quite evident while it did.

* * *

The other admission over that weekend was Theo.

In all my time in the Locked Ward, Theo was one of the patients whose company I enjoyed most. A small man with shoulder-length hair and a goatee beard, he would have been ideal casting for the part of Gimli the dwarf in a remake of *The Lord of the Rings*. He could be the most congenial of company, and made me laugh more than any other person on the ward in all the time I spent there.

I met him at breakfast that first morning. I was in the pantry, doling out breakfast trays from the trolley. He came into the Dayroom, yawning and pushing his hair back from his face. When he came up to the hatch, he looked at me, grinned and pointed.

'Hippy!' he chortled.

'Guilty,' I conceded.

'Me tae!' he whooped with delight. His pleasure was so transparent, you could have seen the distant hills through it. 'What's your name?'

'Dennis.'

'Dennis . . . Dennis . . .?' he mused, as if trying to place me, although he'd never clapped eyes on me before. 'Dennis Hopper!'

'Yeah, man.' I smiled. '*Easy Rider.*'

'*Easy Rider*! Yeah!'

The fact that I had known this made us blood brothers on the instant.

'You're a man with a head full of light!' he chortled again.

I laughed. Luke and Gordon were looking puzzled in the background.

'What's your name?' I asked. 'I need your name to get your breakfast tray.'

'Theo,' he said, suddenly serious. 'And I'm as mad as a spoon.'

Theo was an old hippy, all right. A year or so younger than me, he had dropped out of mainstream society some time in the early 1970s and never been able to find the ladder back up. He clocked me right away as an older version of something similar. We had long conversations about recherché music outfits: the Edgar Broughton Band, Gong, Henry Cow. He suffered from schizophrenia. His delusions were many, but one of them was that he had played in the rock band Black Sabbath, written their hit song 'Paranoid' and had all of his notebooks and songs stolen by Ozzy Osbourne.

I got very fond of Theo and he sensed a kindred spirit, for he attached himself to me very early on. Like many patients, he had absolutely no insight into his condition (despite his joke about being mad as a certain item of cutlery) and he burned with a furious resentment at those he saw as depriving him of his liberty. It was all an Establishment plot by the pigs to hassle him and to do the dirty on all heads and hippies by constantly harshing their mellow and bringing them down.

'I mean, man,' he said to me, 'you should know. You were there in Paris '68. You were at Haight Ashbury. You've seen the pigs in action, man.'

I have no idea why he thought that not only had I hung around with the original hippies in San Francisco, but that I'd also been rioting with the students in Paris, except that he was extremely delusional. If *he* had written 'Paranoid', there was no reason why I should not have torn up the cobblestones with the students at the Sorbonne. *Je suis Marxiste, tendance Groucho.*

He would deliver utterances like this while squatting on his hunkers on the floor next to my seat at the Station.

It was a pose he could hold for hours – no, I mean *hours* – without any ostensible damage to his leg or thigh muscles. If I tried that for ten minutes even, I'd pop a hip. Or at least straighten myself up with all the grace and creak of an ironing board and then limp away like something out of Fellini's *Satyricon*. But Theo must have had the muscle control of a saint on a pillar. Theo Stylites. Or one of those Indian fakirs. He told me that when he was not in hospital he never faced the west in the evening, so that the sun could not set in his eyes.

He considered us to be brothers. He had little time for anybody else. Hunkered there by my seat at the Station, he'd expatiate endlessly on other staff members and how they'd treated him cruelly in the past. It was all fantasy, of course, expressed in terms of the wildest flights of ideas. And Theo never forgot anything. Ever. The smallest incident, the smallest slight, intended or not, was stashed away somewhere in those capacious memory banks. Actually, most of us have equally capacious memories; we just don't have the instant retrieval that Theo had.

'Why you working for a bastard like that weasel Lawlor?' he'd say. (This was Charlie.)

'I don't work *for* him. I work with him.'

'He's a cruel bastard. And he's a pornographer. You know how he makes his money? He makes pornographic movies of his wife with workmen. He makes millions out of prostituting his wife. You know her? She's a nurse too. She works in a medical ward. Lucky for her, because it means she can get the antibiotics she needs to cure herself of all the STDs she gets from fucking strangers for money. Yeah, he's worth millions. You know that restaurant in town, the Jade Pillar? Yeah? Well, he bought that with the money he made from filming his wife fucking anybody and everybody.'

'The Jade Pillar is a Chinese restaurant, Theo.'

'Yeah, and he owns it. How can you be so obtuse, man? You're educated. The bastard's responsible for me being in this fucking predicament in the first place. I was in my pad quite the thing, minding my own business and writing songs, when he came to visit me. And he reported me to the authorities; accused me of having a dog's head in my fridge. And the next thing I know, I'm in the IPCU in that asylum on the hill up there—'

'Hang on, Theo. You had a beheaded dog in your flat?'

He looked at me as if I were a simpleton and then explained slowly and patiently, like a good tutor.

'Well no, man. It was more like a . . . be-dogged head. And it wasn't in the fridge.'

'Why did you have a dog's head in your flat?'

'Somebody gave me it. I'm not into animal cruelty, man, or sacrificing things. But that's not the point. I was arrested in a night raid. The pigs came at night and huckled me out of my place and into the asylum. Then, well, *you* would fight against the forces of evil, wouldn't you, man? Children of the revolution? And because I fought against the brainwashing in there, they arrested me again and threw me in the State Hospital. And the first nurse I met in there was that bastard's brother! Another fucking Lawlor! I couldn't escape them. A vast conspiracy, man.'

The State Hospital is in Carstairs in the Central Belt of Scotland and houses psychiatric patients with tendencies to dangerous, criminal and violent behaviour. It was known widely in the ward as the Big Hoose.

'And Simpson. How can a man of education and culture like you, a man who's read the *Tibetan Book of the Dead*

[I hadn't; I still haven't; I'm not going to], who listens to the Incredible String Band, how can you work with someone like Simpson? He's a thug. A hired thug. He works part-time as a heavy for drug barons in London. I've seen his picture in the papers. I've seen him on the newsreels. He's a torturer. SAS trained. They can never hide it. It's obvious. They bear the mark of Cain. He uses army techniques on patients. I saw him use them in the asylum. He knows all the nerve points. He can paralyse a man in seconds just by sticking his fingers into his neck. That's how they do the big injections. He paralyses the patient and Lawlor injects them with poison.'

Luke was 'a pimp and a rent boy', Clyde 'a poor deluded immigrant forced to work for the services against his will', Gordon 'a moron and an imbecile who'll just do anything the clever ones tell him'. Actually, I agreed with the last bit. But, like Bill, he reserved his greatest bile for Dr Bankstreet.

'That cow, Bankstreet, man. She's an evil bitch. All she wants is to have me incarcerated in here so that I'm not out there in the world. She's terrified I'll tell the newspapers about her. I know all about her injecting folk with mind-altering drugs, man, and getting them to pass on personal secrets. Bank details. Property holdings. All sorts. She has a vault in Switzerland stuffed with Nazi gold and treasure she's extorted through psychic torture. It's all heavy shit, man. She's a fucking witch. The fucking Witch Queen of New Orleans. You know that song, man, don't you?'

'Marie, Marie, da voodoo veau?'

'Yeah, you're hip to the groove. You know, I don't understand why a head like you would want to be working in a torture chamber like this. They were Native Americans, man. Unreconstructed racists call them Red Indians, but the term is Native Americans. You'll know that; you're an educated man. What was it you studied at university?'

'English and American literature.'

'*American* literature, yeah?' He got quite excited. 'Do any Native American literature in that course?'

'Nah. It was all the stuff you'd expect. But I've read some Native American poetry. Gloria Bird. Chrystos. Folk like that.'

'Cool. Yeah, that bitch Bankstreet. She resents me because I'm creative and she's the death force. So she calls me schizophrenic and bangs me up in here, and nobody does anything about it. Do you know, man, she refuses to believe that I wrote Black Sabbath's entire first album? You know the one? With the chick in black by the old watermill on the cover? That's a chick I was balling at the time. I could show you the notebooks, music – well not dots on staves because I'm not into that – just the chords and the lyrics. Lyrics like poetry, man. Like the sublimest poetry, like . . . fucking . . . I don't know . . . Shelley or somebody. I could show you them but Osbourne took all the credit. Nineteen seventy. He's still got my notebooks.'

Most of the time Theo was a gentle kind of a guy. He had been a precocious scholar, brilliant throughout primary and secondary schools. He got six A passes at higher, including English, maths, physics and chemistry. University beckoned. Indeed, he had applied, been accepted and had started on his reading lists when he took ill. Gordon thought he had read too much. That it had turned his brain. Typical of Gordon. Reading did not feature highly in the top ten of Gordon's pastimes. I used to watch him read the red tops in the morning at breakfast, and it wasn't the most edifying sight. I don't mean that he kept a finger under each word as he read and mouthed it to himself. He wasn't quite that bad. It was just obvious that reading a book would have given him a cramp in the brain.

However. A digression. Gordon was of the opinion that too much study had driven Theo mad.

'It's a thin line between genius and madness,' he said.

'A cliché,' said Luke.

'I think the quote you're looking for is Dryden,' I said. '"Great wits are sure to madness near allied".'

'Don't you worry. You're a long way away frae that line,' said John.

Gordon mumped off in a huff. What he said was, as Luke had rightly pointed out, a cliché. And it had no grain of truth in it. The onset of schizophrenia often occurs in late adolescence. That Theo had been an extremely clever young man was just coincidence. The fact that he had begun to smoke dope and experiment with other substances might not have helped.

But that Theo was, far beneath the layers of delusion and paranoia, a clever man was evident to me from the first time we spoke. He knew a great deal about literature, especially the literature that had been trendy at the time of his adolescence. *The Outsider*. *Steppenwolf* – he still had a copy of that. Sometimes, when his mood was more lucid, he asked me questions about writers he liked. He was fond of the work of the Mersey poets: Roger McGough, Adrian Henri and Brian Patten – whom he called with nicely mordant wit, Brain Pattern. He told me that he knew most people considered them a diluted version of the American beats. But, he said, hip though they were, he found those guys 'unreadable'. I agreed with him. Two or three of Ginsberg's poems would do me for all of the beat movement. It was good that somebody like Theo agreed with me.

He had a great interest in science – he had intended to study physics at university. Current scientific developments intrigued him. The Human Genome Project was an obsession. He was greatly exercised by the potentiality of such a breakthrough but, typically, concerned that the result might fall into the hands of the wrong person, some mad Brainiac scientist who would use it to rule the world. And oppress the heads. His interest in the details of the project was much inhibited by his illness. Reading about things of such complexity was now almost totally beyond him. But he knew about its existence.

Mind you, he had devoured the works of Erich von Däniken as well. It figured. Because he was also the New Agest human being I've ever met. If there was anything mystical, occult, paranormal, esoteric, Eastern, pagan or Druid, he was into it.

The first day we met, after he had obviously decided that I was one of the good guys, he came out with a line I truly thought nobody else would ever say to me after 1970.

'Hey, man,' he said, as he passed me on his way to the courtyard, 'what's your sign?'

'Do not disturb,' I rejoined.

It was not original, I have to say, but it seemed singularly appropriate at the time and in the context. Theo thought so too, for he gave a single, sharp bark of amused laughter and kept going. Another time he came into the Dayroom and waved me over to him. He looked excited. He had something clasped tightly in his hand.

'I want you to see something,' he said.

'Okay.'

He stood in front of me and held his hand out, closed. He smiled and nodded his desire that I should extend my hand and receive what he had to reveal. I did. Into my hand he put a small octagonal brown object. It looked like a fossilised chocolate.

'You know what that is?' he asked me.

'Last year's coffee cream?'

He shook his head. 'It's Orgonite.'

'Fancy.'

'You mean you don't know about Orgonite?'

'Well, fuck, don't tell everybody. It might end up in the papers.'

'Orgonite, man. Orgonite.'

'Yeah, I heard you. Orgonite. What the hell is it?'

'Orgonite transforms negative energy into positive, man. It neutralises the pollution from electromagnetic fields. If you conceal it near mobile phone towers and radio masts, it neutralises the negativity. Skies are bluer; grass is greener. It balances the energies of earth and sky, purifies the air and disintegrates rain clouds. Mellows everybody out, man. No bad trips in the vicinity of this baby. If you're troubled by the psychic energy of ley lines, this stuff will groove you out.'

'Well, who isn't troubled by the psychic energy of ley lines?'

'You don't look convinced.'

'Oh, I'm convinced. I'm convinced. I must get some of that Orgonite then. I'm getting a lot of interference on my TV.'

But that was Theo. He believed in, or was interested in, and talked at various times at teeth-gnashing length about,

145

anything and everything hippy-dippy, bohemian or beatnik. He would squat on his hunkers and hold forth at great length, usually while rolling a Rizla.

'Atlantis was like a biblical paradise, you know? The Garden of Eden itself, maybe. Who knows? Animals eating out of the palm of your hand and groovy things like that. No growing old. No suffering. No death.'

'Yeah? What happened in Atlantis, Theo?'

'Well, man, you know, like, it was the world's first civilisation and it was a land of sun worshippers. Beautiful people'.

'Like Ayia Napa?' sneered the passing Gordon.

Theo watched him walk away.

'Fuck! Who is that banana-faced straight? Uncool. Yeah, it was submerged by a tidal wave hundreds of thousands of years ago,' he continued. 'But the really cool thing is this cat, right? He predicted that Atlantis would rise again in 1968 or 1969. It didn't but it could just mean that he miscalculated by twenty or thirty years or something. That would be a trip, right? To see the Garden of Eden, like, float up from the bottom of the sea? And all the cats grooving about, being nice and having fun in the sun.'

'That's from 'Itchycoo Park', isn't it?'

'Yeah, man, that's cool. Good song.'

But the one that I liked most was his yap about Gnosticism. What he actually knew about Gnosticism, I suspect, you could have written on his thumbnail with a fence post. But with this, as with other topics, he talked a good game.

'I'm really into Gnosticism,' he said, apropos of very little at all one afternoon.

'Yeah?'

'Yeah. It's really heavy, you know. It sorts out all that Christian good and evil shit and straightens out your head on it.'

'Sounds like a good idea.'

'Yeah. It's mellow.'

'What's it all about, then, Theo?'

'Well, you know, it's like, this whole world, man, this whole – what would you say? – material world is just a delusion. It's a snare. It's a lure. You know? We are *in* this world at the moment, but not *of* it. Dig? It's all things, man. The soul, the part of us that is above time and this world, this whole plastic scene, is destined for a higher plane. For a fifth dimension. You know, we are one with time and the stars. We are all space travellers. In space and in our heads, man. And the body is just an encumbrance. Just a drag. It doesn't matter what the body does in this world. It's immaterial.'

'I thought you just said it was material. Like the material world.'

'Yeah! Don't fuck with my head, man. You know what I'm saying. Don't be so fucking negative. There's no such thing as sin. Because what the uncool, like, *priest* cats – you know, like that weird Stannie guy – what they call sin is just a whole bunch of things that the body gets up to in this world. It can't touch the soul. The soul is away on a different plane and just longing for immersion into the One. That's what uncool dudes can't fathom. You know? Like religious zeroes. That's why it's sound to be a head. Like I am. And maybe you, man, if you didn't work in this fucking prison! Because that's where it's happening. That's where the soul is. You know? You can feed and water the body and let it do what it wants. But the soul needs thoughts and dreams and music and poetry and love. And they go in at the head. You've got to feed the head.'

'That's 'White Rabbit', isn't it?'

Theo laughed.

'Fuck off, man. So what if it's 'White Rabbit'? The whole universe is a battleground of good and evil, and the soul is on the side of the good guys. Let your body do what it feels like. It can't alter anything. It's just, like, the means of transport that gets our heads from A to B. You know?'

He straightened up and walked away. I think I had offended him. I can't fully itemise all the half-baked and semi-digested religious and philosophical offcuts that went into that particular swill bucket of a theory but I can tell you one thing. Gnosticism it most assuredly was gnot.

19

Cupid is a knavish lad,
Thus to make poor females mad.
William Shakespeare,
A Midsummer Night's Dream

Winter came to the ward and the world. Starting at 7.30 in the morning and finishing at 8.30 at night, I rose in the dark and drove home in the dark. In morning's smoky blue darkness, lit by the distant rose of street lights, I scraped the car windscreen. In evening's jet black, lit by the lights of the hospital, looking like a liner in the sea of night, I scraped it again. Sleet spattered the long windows of the Dayroom as the patients ate or watched TV. The wind grew honed and serious as a switchblade. Patients who had occasionally wandered out into the courtyard for their smoke, even through the autumn weeks, now settled for the warm fug of the Smoke Room. Only Voytek, happed up in his greatcoat like a downcast Polish officer, sometimes stood stock still in a corner of the yard and smoked his roll-ups as the light faded and the barometer fell.

From four o'clock every afternoon some of the ward lights were turned on. It gave the place a dim and romantic glow, alternate pools of light and shadow down the long central corridor, wan reflections through the glass panels of the Pool Room walls into the Dayroom. Outside, the lights flickered on around the car park, like a scatter of change.

Then snow began to fall, drifting slowly down from the sky, grey gone gold as it sprayed through the lamplight, strange and momentary moths against the dark glass of the windows. The world cramped down and crept in close around the ward. Now the one or two stragglers making their way through the hospital grounds towards the car parks were black smudges in the whirling landscape. It was remarkably and remotely beautiful as if the night, the snow and the hospital were a world in a colossal paperweight.

And as the snow and frost covered the land, we had two admissions, one after the other, in very quick succession. Both were female and both had been badly treated by love.

The first was a woman in her late thirties, very tall, slim and with short bright-red hair. Norma was an air hostess. She had been having an affair with a married pilot. When his wife found out, she demanded that he immediately jettison the cargo, if he wanted to remain married and be with his family. Notwithstanding the fact that he had sworn to Norma many times that *she* was the one he truly loved and wanted to be with, and that he would finish with his wife the minute that . . . whatever he promised, whatever these guys always promise . . . despite all that, as soon as Mrs Pilot issued her ultimatum, he acceded to all her demands and grounded himself.

Norma had a crisis, during which she attempted to take her own life with an overdose of prescription sleeping pills. It didn't mean anything to her that she was a player in a clichéfied love story; she loved the unfaithful double-dealing bastard. She had believed him when he told her he would divorce his wife so he and Norma could set up home in Rose Coloured Cottage by the Lake of Dreams and be happy ever after. You and I know it's the old, old story, but that's only because we are not involved in it. When you're in your own love story, you believe in it, no matter how preposterous the setting or how unlikely the characterisation.

She came to us from a hospital in the city. She had been admitted there after her suicide attempt and had seemed on the mend. But she made another attempt on her life and was transferred out to us. She meant it. She didn't want to live without her lover – spineless and insincere as he was.

I felt sorry for Norma. She was a good person; she had just had the bad luck to love the wrong man. She made another serious attempt on her life a few days after she arrived in 25 and started on a course of meds. Ursula called her for breakfast, watched as she rose, collected her things and went into the shower. In there, she tried to strangle herself with her tights. Fortunately, Ursula, being an experienced nurse, sensed something was wrong and dashed in without knocking. Norma was slumped at the foot of the wall, still in her PJs, with her tights round her neck and attached to the door handle. She was crimson in the face. It took two people to dig the tights out of the flesh on her neck.

She was specialed after that. And I have to say that my female colleagues did a superb job, sitting with her, talking, listening, letting her unburden herself of all the emotions seething inside her. Anger. Resentment. Betrayal. Hurt. Many more. After a couple of days they had Norma smiling – a thin, watery ghost of a smile, granted, but a vast improvement on the grim motionless face she'd arrived with. A few days after that, she was laughing.

I've no doubt that the girls started off by telling her that all men are bastards, not just her lover. None of them worth it. Arrant knaves, all. Believe none of them. But they didn't stop there; they were far better than that. Passing by where Norma sat in the Dayroom with one of them, we could see her reacting better every day to company. They would be talking about what was in the news, or what was on TV, sharing stories of family life. Common or garden life. Norma slowly started to thrive on it. We could see it in the smile she greeted us with at the hatch, or the way she answered when we asked how she was doing.

And then her sense of humour started to show itself. And it was a good one.

'You're looking well, Norma.'

'Yeah. One thing about being dumped by a lying two-faced louse and then going into a depression, the weight just falls off you. I can recommend it. The Other Woman Diet.'

'Looking good on it, at least. Biscuit with that coffee?'

'No fear. Not now. If I lose another stone, I could get the air chief marshal to chuck his wife for me.'

I liked that.

A week later Norma was transferred back to the city hospital and discharged from there within a few days. I've heard nothing of her since. I hope she's happy. She deserves it. Hell, everybody deserves at least that.

The festive period was upon us. The females unearthed a box of old decorations and fairy lights, and an artificial tree that had originally been pressed into service about the time the Magi left Bethlehem. They spent a fun-filled afternoon pinning up shiny tinsel bells, draping streamers in loops and in festoons on walls and from ceilings, trimming the tree with paste balls, jamming the pointy top of the tree through the arse of an entirely blameless fairy and then trying to get the lights to work. They couldn't.

'Do you know anything about Christmas lights, Dennis?'

'Nope.'

'You don't sound very Christmassy.'

'It's not Christmas. It's December the twelfth. I like to wassail as much as the next man, but at Christmas. Not for weeks before it. I hate the way Christmas starts in August nowadays. You can't drive home from October but some new wazzock every day is putting those bloody fairy lights up on his roof. I mean, if the idea is that Christmas is a wonderful time for a couple of days, don't you think you kinda waste the effect by having everywhere covered with that shit from a month before it?'

'It's just people being jolly and friendly.'

'No, it isn't. It's cheap tat. It's – wouldn't you know it? – American. I blame television and the movies. If it's American, it's got to be good. Bollocks. Have you never noticed how kids don't go guising any more? They go trick or treating. It's the same basic notion, but 'guising' was the Scottish term. 'Trick or treat' is American. It's completely taken over, like the fucking grey squirrel. Kids don't hollow out tumshies any more for turnip lanterns. They get a pumpkin from the fucking supermarket. A pumpkin! God alfuckinmighty! When was the last time anybody round here ever ate a pumpkin?'

'Kinna losin' it a bit now, Dennis.'

'Yeah. Pam, draw one up for him and jag him in the jacksie.'

'And no, I don't know anything about fairy lights.'

'Luke! You any good with Christmas lights?'

'I'll try.'

'Thanks. Ebenezer here doesn't like Christmas.'

'I do like fucking Christmas. I just like it at Christmas *time*!'

'Bah humbug.'

'Cliché! But you can call me Herod.'

Luke fixed the lights. They rigged them up. It looked okay. If you like that kind of thing. Then they found a small fibre-optic tree at the bottom of the cupboard. They set that up too. It sat on the window sill, flickering its multicoloured branch-tips at everybody. You couldn't sit and watch the TV without kaleidoscopic waves of tiny dots flashing in the periphery of your vision. How I loved it.

Theo sauntered in, clocked it and enthused. 'Far out, man! A tripping tree!'

I have to say that in the evening, with most of the Dayroom lights out, the effect was quite atmospheric. Santa's psycho grotto, as Theo called it.

Cordelia joined us the week before Christmas. Love was the source of her problems too. But hers was a much more unusual and complicated case than Norma's had been.

She was a delightful young woman who spoke with the clipped vowels of the city's educated middle class. (The fact that she was called Cordelia was another clue as to her origins. There were no wee girls named after Shakespearean tragic heroines in my primary school. No Desdemona McGroarty, or Ophelia O'Flaherty.) She was in her twenties, extremely bright, intelligent and gregarious, and extremely good-looking. She also had something of the bohemian about her. Tie-dye tops or tunic dresses with jeans. Pinafore dresses. Harem trousers or cotton leggings printed in swirling colours. Huge earrings. Sandals. An air of candles and crystals. She said she could read palms and do tarot readings. (Theo fell in love with her on the instant.) She was bubbly and vivacious and enchanting company. There was always the faint zing of finger cymbals when she appeared. Or maybe that was just me.

Her problem was that she was obsessively in love with one of the GPs at her local surgery.

This was an older man, and a happily married one with a family, who entertained not the slightest notion for her. She was just one of his patients. He treated her with the courtesy and professionalism with which he treated any other patient. As you would expect. But she had mistaken this for simmering and barely restrained ardour. She took to haunting his surgery like lovesick ectoplasm. At least once a week she tried to make an appointment to see him. If she couldn't get him and was offered another doctor, she was far from gruntled.

Being a man of some insight, Doc began to realise that there was more to Cordelia than just a plethora of minor complaints like bunions and vague gastric trouble. He suggested hypochondria might really be her problem. But he suggested it so kindly that she knew he was desperately in love with her.

I can't remember exactly what the next imaginary illness was that she presented herself with at the clinic, but it might have been respiratory difficulty of some kind or possibly a lump in her breast. Whatever it was, it gave her the opportunity of removing her top for examination. The doctor, being a wise man and somewhat schooled in the ways of the world, asked Cordelia to remove her top when he was out of the room, fetching a female colleague to ride shotgun on the examination.

When he returned in the company of a female practice nurse, Cordelia was completely naked. She offered her favours to the hapless doc. He understandably made himself scarce on the instant. The nurse roared at Cordelia to get dressed at once, and threw her her clothes. Cordelia didn't quite understand the meaning of what had happened. She was of the opinion that the object of her desire had fled because of the presence of the nurse, and that, if she had not been there, he would have cast himself with glee upon her. He was consumed with lust for her. She knew that.

The nurse had said no, he wasn't.

Cordelia had said yes, he was.

The nurse had said he was old enough to be her father; he had a wife and children; he was happily married.

Cordelia had said *that* meant nothing at all. She knew he loved *her*, not his wife.

The nurse had said how the hell did she know that the doctor loved her?

Cordelia had said because she recognised the secret signals.

That was the point at which the nurse and the doctor, who was having a skulk in the corridor outside, knew that they were dealing with someone who had become badly unhinged. The doctor, assured that Cordelia was now dressed, came back into the room and tried, kindly, to disabuse her of the delusion that he had any feelings for her. Cordelia was having none of it. She said she knew that if the nurse were not there he would be happy to go down on one knee and plight his troth.

The long and the short of the ensuing scene was that Cordelia lost it altogether and ran amok, scattering papers, pen, keyboard, stethoscope and assorted other medical stuff from the doctor's desk, howling and shrieking, rending her garments and tearing her hair out in lumps. More Cassandra than Cordelia, really. She was sectioned and removed to the hospital in the city. She wasn't detained there long; fairly soon she was discharged. But she didn't help her case any. Somehow or other she found out the doc's home address and phone number. She took to sending him long rambling letters declaring her undying passion for him and, no doubt, urging him to ride up on a white charger some night to a spot below her window, from where he could rescue her. She left messages of love on his voicemail. She left little presents on his doorstep at dawn. Love tokens. Nothing out of the ordinary. Nothing so vulgar as pearls in wine, or the head of John the Baptist. Just flowers and poems and little trinkets. He went to the law. Cordelia was served with a restraining order – an injunction, a non-molestation order – something that prevented her from bugging the doc. It was obvious now what Cordelia's illness was. Erotomania.

Called 'unrequited love' for centuries, and often confused with nymphomania or satyriasis, this is a condition whereby the sufferer believes that another person is in love with them. But not someone who actually *is* in love with them – a husband, wife, girlfriend or boyfriend – rather, a total stranger. Sometimes a celebrity the sufferer has developed a fixation on. It is a psychotic symptom, since it is completely delusional and can be symptomatic of schizophrenia or bipolar illness. The sufferer is convinced that the object of his or her affections returns the feeling and communicates the regard in covert ways, such as secret signals, meaningful glances and other forms of coded behaviour. These might be increasingly baroque and detached from reality, such as the way the person's curtains are arranged or the clothes he or she wears on a particular day. The sufferer, however, demonstrates his or her love by overt means, such as Cordelia did – phone calls, letters, presents and visits. It used to be called (and still is in some quarters) 'de Clérambault's syndrome' after the French psychiatrist who researched it. It is not to be confused with the phenomenon of stalking, which is part of a separate condition known as Obsessive Love. That is a potentially more dangerous condition that follows a distinct pattern of events and reactions.

After the doctor took out the injunction against her, she stopped phoning and writing to him but took to driving by his house at random times of the day and night. Then to walking past it. Then to standing in the bushes of someone else's garden on the opposite side of the road from his driveway so that she could see him leave for work in the morning.

Finally, she made one last desperate throw of the dice. One sunny afternoon, when she knew he would be in surgery sawing bones and dispensing tablets, she boldly walked up his drive and rang his doorbell. When Mrs Doc answered the door, Cordelia told her that she was the daughter of one of the doc's university friends. Her name was Elsie Drummond and she lived in Dublin nowadays but was just passing through the city after a conference and thought she might just take a chance and look up her dad's old student chum. Was she being a nuisance?

Well, Mrs Doc had never seen Cordelia and didn't know Elsie Drummond from El Cid. But she was shrewd. She had an idea of who this young woman was. No, of course Elsie wasn't being a nuisance. Alistair would be delighted to see her. Why didn't she come in and they could have a nice cup of tea? She was all middle class and frightfully terribly absolutely.

Cordelia was taken into the shrine, and Mrs Doc went away and made a nice cup of tea and they sat in the conservatory and had a lovely time. Cordelia was all eyes at a banquet, drinking in every detail of the house, the furnishings and the photographs. Was that their oldest? My, what a good-looking girl. At school in the city? Private school, of course. Absolutely, one must maintain standards and where are you going to get standards in the comprehensive system?

Then the house door opened and the doc's voice called, 'Hello.'

That was when Cordelia began to scent a large brown rodent. Mrs Doc had phoned her husband while she was ostensibly in the kitchen making tea. Needless to say, he knew nothing of any young woman called Elsie Drummond and had no friends of university days with daughters who might be living in Ireland. On the other hand . . .

There was a scene, of course. He ordered Cordelia from his property and threatened once again to have recourse to the law. Cordelia exited as scornfully as she could, her head held high. The door was slammed behind her and she had no doubt he was phoning the law or the hospital even then. She knew it was all the wife's fault – she could see the cunning and conniving bitch at the picture window. So she flicked a double set of Vs at her, mooned and then made good her flight.

She looked slightly shamefaced when she told me that.

'You did that? It doesn't seem at all like you.'

'I did, yes. It was a frightfully vulgar thing to do, I know. But, well, that vulgar bism was looking out the window at me with a look of triumph. And I thought, "Right, lady, we'll soon see about you!" So I gave her the fingers. And a flash of my backside.'

'I don't know that I approve but I certainly understand. I'd never have pegged you, though, as the girl to do anything like that.'

'Well, nor would I,' she said, aghast at the very idea. 'Normally. But circumstances alter cases. Isn't that what they say?'

'I shouldn't be at all surprised,' I said.

'Anyway, he doesn't want to be with her any more. He doesn't love her; he loves me.'

'But, if he threw you out of the house . . .'

'That was only because *she* was there. That much is obvious. He couldn't make love to me with her there.'

'But he threw you out of the surgery too.'

'Well, *that* was because the nurse was there!'

She got a little snappy then, which wasn't like her, so I back-pedalled a bit on the rational enquiries.

'How do you know he loves you?'

'Little things. Little things that only a lover would pick up on. When the lounge light is on, it means that she's at home and he has to go through the motions. Being a husband and father.'

'Right.'

'But when the top bedroom window is open at night, with the curtains drawn, that means he wants to see me in the near future. A window of opportunity.'

'Right. It couldn't just be that they want some fresh air in the bedroom at night?'

'Don't be so prosaic, Dennis.'

'Oh, sorry. I'll try not to be. Does he leave you any other signs?'

'There was one morning I went through the bins. He had left a copy of the paper, turned to a certain page. The main story on that page was about the most popular boys' and girls' names in Scotland over the last ten years or so. That was a sign.'

'Yeah? Were the top names Alistair and Cordelia?'

'No, they were Jack and Chloe, actually. But it showed me that he wanted us to start a family ourselves.'

Nothing could persuade Cordelia that these were entirely delusional beliefs. The signs were as real and as meaningful to her as any lover's letter or token was to – well, 'normal', lovers. 'The lunatic, the lover, and the poet, are of imagination all compact,' as Shakespeare says. The thing that fascinated me about her was that it was only in this one regard that her behaviour was in any way abnormal. She was university educated and highly intelligent. Brainy as brain soup. She worked in the university library in the city and was stimulating company for an old literature buff like myself. We blethered for ages about writers and works. Cordelia was especially interested in women's writing and extremely knowledgeable about people like Virginia Woolf, Iris Murdoch and Beryl Bainbridge. I told her Iris Murdoch was a favourite writer of mine and we spent a day in deep discussion of her novels. Cordelia was interested in my championing of Jeanette Winterson as one of the finest stylists of our age. I found her fascinating company.

She was quite open in our conversations. One day, escorting her to the shop (she was allowed time out from an early date), I was curious to find out more about her.

'Do you mind if I ask you something, Cordelia?' I said as we strolled along.

'No.'

'You might think I'm impertinent, or that it's too personal.'

'I'll tell you if I do.'

'Okay. You're not married, are you?'

'Married? No. Never met Mr Right. Well, actually, I did once. I went out for a while with a teacher called Frank Wright – not Frank Lloyd Wright, just Frank Wright. But he wasn't really Mr Right. With an R. Just Mr Wright with a Wuh. So, no.'

'Well, have you ever had a relationship with a man? You know what I mean . . . I mean a long-term or meaningful relationship, I suppose.'

'You mean have I had sexual relationships before? Oh yes. Oh dear me, yes. You forget I was a student. And I was slimmer then.'

'You're hardly a hippo now.'

'No, I mean I was quite attractive.'

'You're attractive now.'

'Oh well, so far as that goes. Yes. That's nice of you to say. But when I was younger . . . I was good-looking.'

I didn't correct her. I not only meant that she was a very attractive personality – which she undoubtedly was – I also meant that she was very attractive physically. And vivacious, as I said. But I felt that to go on about that would have been to alter the emphasis of what I meant to talk about and might even verge on the creepy. So I didn't. But I'd got the information I was interested in. She was able to form relationships, of some depth and significance, with people in the conventional way. She hadn't lived her life imagining that a taxi driver, or a holiday guide, say, had formed an intense and burning love for her when all he had been doing was being nice as he did his job.

'I wasn't just talking about sexual relationships. Have you been in love before? With a man who loved you?'

'Oh yes. Yes, of course. We all have, haven't we?'

In the literature on erotomania there are references to lonely and introverted people who feel unloved and, as a result, become deluded that people like doctors, nurses, dentists, social workers or church volunteers – anyone liable to be compassionate and caring in their working lives – have fallen in love with them. Cordelia – young, bright, gregarious – was hardly a textbook case. But then, as I was rapidly finding out, there was no such thing as a textbook case.

Dr Bankstreet prescribed a common atypical antipsychotic. Cordelia complied with the meds, stayed on the ward for the time it took, and was one of the most pleasant and personable characters ever to grace its confines. When she was transferred back to the city hospital, I was sorry to see her go – not for her sake, but in a purely selfish way. She'd been somebody quite, quite different. A rare and exotic visitor to our shore.

As with so many others, I heard no more of her when she left. That might be a good thing. It might mean that she'd been cured of her obsession with her GP, that she wasn't liable to be found on his lawn at night, pawing the grass and howling at the moon. Or mooning at his wife, for that matter.

20

Be patient; for I will not let him stir
Till I have used the approved means I have,
With wholesome syrups, drugs and holy prayers,
To make of him a formal man again:
William Shakespeare, *The Comedy of Errors*

Okay. Up to now, here and there I have referred to medication used in the treatment of various patients. This is not a learned treatise on psychiatric medicine, but I should pause to discuss meds briefly here. For anyone more deeply interested, there is much literature on the subject. This is the briefest outline of what I learned on the ward. A skitter through the main points. And, if you're not interested, now's the time to flick to the next chapter.

The first thing to note is that medication is only one method of treatment among many available to psychiatrists. Significant advances are also made by several other kinds of therapy.

Everybody knows the cliché of a patient lying back on a couch while a psychoanalyst sits on a leather chair by him, legs crossed, taking notes. This is a simplified picture of psychoanalysis. The patient is urged to speak freely and let his mind wander. The analyst then interprets the patient's stories and helps him identify underlying psychological problems that they could work to resolve. Sceptical colleagues of Freud called this the 'talking cure', and it was based on his belief that, in the words of an old TV commercial, 'It's good to talk.' Shakespeare certainly thought so. 'Give sorrow words,' as Malcolm tells Macduff; 'the grief that does not speak, / Whispers the o'er fraught heart and bids it break.' Psychoanalysis is still in use.

Cognitive Behaviour Therapy (CBT) is a combination, unsurprisingly, of cognitive and behavioural therapies. Psychiatrists noticed during some sessions of psychoanalysis that patients did not report some very deep thoughts which often prompted extreme emotions. CBT is designed to retrieve these thoughts, then address them and the behaviour they prompt, so easing the patient towards improvement. If you remove the symptoms, the thinking goes, you remove the disorder.

Family Therapy emphasises close relationships between family members as a significant factor in helping someone get better. The concern and attention of loved ones can be a major contribution to stabilising a condition and recovery from it.

There are other therapies. Counselling can give people support and information to help them understand and manage their problems. It was what the staff on our ward did on a daily basis. Psychoeducation courses provide the opportunity for people with mental illnesses to study their condition, understand it and help them cope. The theory is, if you understand what's happening to you, you know better how to deal with it. Self-help groups, supported accommodation and peer support programmes do the same thing.

Creative therapies, such as Music or Art Therapy, can increase judgement and insight through the creative process while relieving stress, improving mood and enhancing social skills. And ECT, electroconvulsive therapy, as I mentioned earlier, has remarkable success rates in certain cases.

But yes, medication is a significant part of psychiatric treatment. Pharmacotherapy. Let me make it plain here that I never prescribed or administered any medicines at any time. That was all done by the clever folk. The ones who knew what they were doing. But if you work with people long enough, you eventually notice what they're doing, and the things they're doing it with. So, an interested observer's take on psychiatric meds:

There are several categories including antidepressants, anxiolytics, mood stabilisers and antipsychotics.

Antidepressants (uppers), fairly obviously, work to counteract depression. They increase wakefulness, alertness and motivation. In the 1950s it was common to prescribe opioids as antidepressants. Although primarily painkillers, a noted side effect of these drugs was sedation. In the 1960s amphetamines, known to increase wakefulness and focus, were used. Both opioids and amphetamines work extremely quickly, showing positive results in twenty-four hours or, at most, forty-eight. Modern antidepressants work by targeting certain chemicals in the brain, most notably serotonin, a biochemical known to assist in feelings of well-being. There are many classes of these drugs and a multitude of brand names.

Anxiolytics (downers, formerly called minor tranquillisers) reduce anxiety. Perhaps the best known are the benzodiazepines (benzos). They are used to combat anxiety both in the short and long terms and are used as a first choice for short-term sedation. The best known drugs in this class are diazepam and lorazepam. We called lorazepam 'blues' on the ward. Something to do with the colour, I think. Barbiturates, formerly prescribed for anxiety, are hardly ever prescribed now, on account of the risks of abuse and addiction. Some herbs are said to have anxiolytic qualities – St John's wort, valerian, golden root and catnip, for example. We never used them. Pity. It might have been nice to watch Pamela or Clyde dispense simples from the meds trolley, like the wise one in a medieval village.

Mood stabilisers are used to treat mood-swing conditions like bipolar disorder. Anticonvulsants, used in the treatment of epilepsy, such as sodium valproate and lamotrigine, have mood stabilising properties and were used on the ward. But the classic mood stabilising drug was the most commonly used on 25: lithium. (This is not to be confused with *di*lithium, which we never used, since its crystals could be used to power the patient's warp drive system and project him to the farthest edge of the universe.)

Antipsychotics treat the major psychotic illnesses, and symptoms like delusions, hallucinations and disordered thought. They fall into two main categories.

The first generation of antipsychotic drugs were also known as 'typical' antipsychotics, and psychiatry came upon them almost by chance. Chlorpromazine, for example, was developed originally as a surgical anaesthetic and was then discovered to have powerful calmative effects when patients awoke. It was prescribed for psychiatric patients and considered a chemical improvement on lobotomy. (Lobotomy consisted of surgery on part of the brain's frontal lobes. Developed as a treatment in the 1930s to calm violently aggressive patients, it continued to be routinely used for over twenty-five years. The fact that it had grave and consistent side effects made little difference.)

So chlorpromazine was seen as a boon. It was still used in the Locked Ward. Other first-generation antipsychotics still in use in 25 included haloperidol, depixol and clopixol acuphase. A patient who was aggressive might be given 'two blues and a larry' or 'two and five' – a dose of two milligrams of lorazepam and five of haloperidol to sedate him in the short term and reduce his tendency to aggression in the longer run. (The nickname 'larry' came from a shortened form of the first-generation brand name Largactil.) A patient who showed a tendency to increased violence, or violence on a regular scale, might be given an injection of clopixol acuphase, for acute sedation.

Second-generation or 'atypical' antipsychotics, like their predecessors, target a neurochemical substance called dopamine. Dopamine plays an important part in aspects of an individual's personality like behaviour, motivation, mood and attention. Atypical antipsychotics regularly prescribed on 25 included clozapine, olanzapine, risperidone, quetiapine and amisulpride.

Antipsychotics can have serious side effects, none more so than clozapine's potential to cause leukopenia (a reduction in the number of white cells in the blood). But all powerful drugs have side effects. The known side effects of first-generation antipsychotics include muscular spasms of the neck, jaw, tongue or eyes; tremor in the limbs while resting; involuntary and repetitive body movements, and an inability to sit still or remain motionless. Some of these may be reduced or even absent with second-generation antipsychotics, but equally they may still be present. Other side effects of second-generation antipsychotics include sexual dysfunction, diabetes, pronounced weight gain and even lowered life expectancy. They are what one patient called 'heavy shit'.

The whole topic of drugs, particularly antipsychotics, in psychiatry is a controversial one. Some professionals question the success of these medications, doubting whether they actually *treat* psychosis. They suggest that drugs are a form of chemical control, a way of making difficult patients manageable. Since they tend to make patients calmer, there is the danger, say some, that they might be overused to make life easier for everyone else.

I don't know enough about these things to be able to take sides. I can only say that I saw our patients treated with a variety of medications and also saw improvements.

A PRN medication was often prescribed. The letters come from the Latin phrase *pro re nata*. This means 'as the thing happens', and it was also called 'as-required' medication. It was a med that the patient could ask for, when he or she felt she needed it. Benzos were commonly prescribed as PRN meds, to help patients cope with anxiety.

One final word. I have referred to the difficulty that psychie staff commonly experience with patients' non-compliance with drug taking. Some tactics help, like prescribing liquid forms where available, or the increasing use of velotabs, thin film-like tablets that dissolve in the mouth, so that hiding under the tongue makes no difference; the drug is absorbed in any case. But the most effective method of tackling patient reluctance – or forgetfulness – is the depot injection. The drug in a depot injection is in an oil suspension so that it is released gradually over a long period of time. A depot might be administered every week, fortnight or month. So, with the reduction in the frequency of dosing, compliance is vastly improved and the drug is released into the body consistently over the prescribed time.

21

*. . . he on honey-dew hath fed
And drunk the milk of Paradise.*

Samuel Taylor Coleridge, 'Kubla Khan'

Meanwhile, on a matter not a million miles removed . . .

It became increasingly obvious to me that a substantial number of admissions related to what the medical staff called 'drug-induced psychoses'. At one point, every week or two at most, some young person would be admitted who was orbiting the planet Neptune because some chemical they had ingested was doing weird things to their brains. Mostly, though not exclusively, young men in their twenties, they were climbing the walls when they were admitted. They often had to be restrained from attempting the climb again when in the ward. The north face of the Dayroom wall was a particular favourite. Perhaps they tried to climb it simply because it was there. Although, truth to tell, it was hard to make out just what was 'there' for some of these young men. Whatever the chemical they had taken, it had melted the distinction between the real and the imaginary for many of them.

It's quite disturbing to watch someone with a fit of the screaming habdabs, so by implication a lot worse for the poor bastard undergoing it. I've seen them gibbering in the corner of an Interview Room, cowering in a fetal position, arms wrapped protectively around the head. I've seen them look upon thin air and their eyes widen in abject terror at whatever horror was rising from the space/time continuum to overwhelm them. I've seen them lash out wildly at swarming hallucinations. Drug-induced psychoses are just as real – or unreal – as any other, just as incapacitating, just as terrifying, but brought on by some drug the patient has taken for recreational purposes. They weren't deriving a lot of recreation from them by the time they arrived on the ward.

It is useful to make a distinction at this point. Psychosis can be *induced* by drugs or can be assisted or worsened by them. Some drugs, like amphetamines, can actually *cause* psychosis; some drugs, like cannabis, can trigger psychosis in someone who is vulnerable. And, for anyone who has experienced psychosis, the risks of taking street drugs for recreational purposes are even higher. Another factor to be considered is that antipsychotic medication can react powerfully with some street drugs and alcohol.

The symptoms of drug-induced psychoses are just the same as for any other psychosis – hallucinations, delusions, paranoia, extreme anxiety, mania, grandiosity and increased aggression. Other unpleasantnesses brought on by misuse of drugs include formication, which is a freaky sensation of insects crawling all over the skin or, even freakier, *under* it. This is so common a symptom that it has been nicknamed 'cocaine bugs'. 'Tweaking' is the nickname given to repeated, almost uncontrollable, movements like swaying, rocking or crossing and uncrossing legs that the sufferer of a drug-induced psychosis might find himself afflicted with. The treatment is often an antipsychotic like haloperidol or olanzapine.

Skoosh was a twenty-something guy with a crystal meth habit when he was brought in handcuffs to 25 by the police. He had threatened an elderly GP in a local surgery when off his tits on what he called 'ice'. (When I was at university the common nickname for it was 'speed'. There are a variety of others.) People take it because it gives them a powerful rush – a sudden surge of euphoria – as well as increased energy levels and sex drive. Conversely, it can make the taker paranoid, agitated and confused. It is also wickedly addictive.

Skoosh was wild when the police brought him in, threatening all sorts of mayhem to everyone in the Interview Room the minute his cuffs were removed. So they weren't. A male SHO was interviewing him; the two policemen who brought him in were present and so was John. Luke and I lurked outside in the corridor as backup. The SHO repeatedly asked him what he had taken; Skoosh repeatedly threatened to 'kick his cunt in' whenever he was freed. He stood up from his chair at one point and made a lunge at the doc. John huckled him back into his seat and then restrained him from moving any further. Skoosh said he would kick *his* cunt in, the minute the opportunity for such a kicking presented itself. The SHO tried again to find out exactly how much, of exactly what, Skoosh had taken. Skoosh made the usual threat, so the SHO decided that perhaps an intra-muscular injection of two blues and a larry would restore to Skoosh the equanimity he lacked at that point.

Also at that point he asked the policemen to remove the bracelets that were causing Skoosh so much unhappiness. They did, and Skoosh went for it. He breenged again, only this time at John, his fists and feet flying. Luke and I tore into the room. However, John and two policemen were more than enough to restrain him. They had him down on the floor in the classic position in a jiffy. Maybe less; maybe half a jiffy. It's difficult to judge the size of jiffies. As the

SHO left to draw up the jag, Luke and I took over from the policemen. It's easy. Mirroring the exact position of the man you are relieving, you slide in behind and carefully replace his person with your own. Then the police, having other pressing matters in hand, left. The while, Skoosh was loudly threatening the severest damage to everyone's female genitalia with his feet.

He was jagged and, after ten or fifteen minutes, had subsided sufficiently for us to remove the restraint and stand up. We escorted him to his room and let him sleep it off.

Next morning he was a sorry sight. Shivering and obsessively grinding his teeth, he shambled into the Treatment Room for morning meds. In response to Geraldine's question as to how he was feeling, he replied, 'Rattling.' By which he meant he had a hollow feeling in his gut, felt drained and lifeless and had a dose of the jitters.

'You've certainly got the Charlie Drakes,' said John, nodding at Skoosh's violently shaking hands.

'Aye.'

'Must be a good rush, to make all that shit worthwhile,' observed John.

Skoosh just shivered and shook his head. What would John know about that?

It turned out that Skoosh had been a heroin user in the past and had managed to get himself off of that spectral merry-go-round, which was an impressive achievement by anybody's standards. He still had the urge for a chemical high, though. Dope, speed, Es – anything would serve his purpose when the maggot bit him.

'Cannae understand that kind a mentality,' mused John over breakfast one morning.

'What kind of mentality?' said Rona.

'The one that makes you take drugs.'

'Drugs like nicotine?' said Rona.

'That's different,' snorted John, a smoker.

'Drugs like alcohol?' said Rona.

John shook his head dismissively. 'Different aw thegither.'

'They cause more damage than any other drug,' said Rona.

'How? How do they?'

'They cost society more than all the illegal drugs combined,' said Rona.

'After heroin and cocaine,' pointed out Charlie, 'it's alcohol and tobacco. In terms of what's most dangerous to the user. Rona's point might just be right about what they cost society.'

'You never taken anything?' Luke asked John.

'Drugs? Never. You?'

'Smoked a bit of dope,' Luke admitted.

'You, Dennis?'

'I used to be a hippy, remember.'

'Used to be?' sneered Gordon.

'I think dope is different,' mused Luke.

'Could make you experiment with other drugs,' said Rona.

'There's little evidence for that,' said Charlie. 'In fact, it's interesting. Most hard drug users started on dope. But it isn't the case that most people who smoke dope go on to hard drugs.'

This gave Gordon pause, a semi-breve rest to be precise. You could see he was having trouble with it. Before he could articulate his semantic quandary, however, Luke spoke.

'I could see why you might want to try smoking dope. Or taking an E. Or quite a lot of things. But heroin? That's the one that puzzles me. At what point in the process of tying a tourniquet onto your arm, tapping up a vein and jabbing a syringe full of shit into your bloodstream, do you think to yourself – "I'm only going to try this once. No matter how good the high, I'm not going to get addicted. I'm no going to be like all they junkies that couldn't handle it." Surely the odds must be obvious to you?'

'Ah,' said Charlie, 'that's how *you* think about it. Different mindset altogether.'

Luke was in the pantry at lunchtime, doling out the tuck. I was footering in the background, making myself a coffee or assisting in some other way, when Skoosh came up to the hatch.

'Could I have a soup spoon, please?'

'What?' said Luke.

'This spoon,' said Skoosh, holding it up. 'They sent me this spoon for my soup. But it's a dessert spoon. Look.'

Luke regarded Skoosh and the spoon for three seconds, then silently took the offending item from him and replaced it with a soup spoon. Skoosh said thanks and went away.

'Well, that'll fuckin' do me,' said Luke. 'Doesn't mind chokin' the life out of some poor auld doctor an' trashin' his surgery when he's junked up on crystal meth; doesn't mind shootin' up, but he cannae take his soup wi' a fuckin' dessert spoon.'

'A man's got to have standards,' I said.

'He'd a used it five years ago for cookin' up his works,' snarled Luke. 'Wouldn't have bothered his arse if it was round or sharp then, eh?'

Luke was not usually a sneerer, but he had some issues with people who took up beds because they, as he put it, 'couldnae handle their drug of choice'. He wasn't the only one.

While most cases of drug-induced psychosis arose as a result of taking what are commonly known as hard drugs, such as cocaine, heroin, LSD and so on, one or two were associated with the regular and heavy use of cannabis. Medical science has known for some time that it is a dangerous mistake to call cannabis a soft drug. The evidence is increasingly persuasive as regards cognitive impairment (sometimes permanent) and development of psychosis arising from the use of cannabis. Cannabis can cause irreversible damage to the brain, and it seems that the brains of teenagers are particularly susceptible.

The problem is worsened because most of the cannabis available today is much more powerful than the stuff that was available in my day. These more powerful strains (commonly known as skunk) contain a higher proportion of tetrahydrocannabinol (THC, the main psychoactive ingredient, which has analgesic properties but is also thought to induce psychosis), and far less of the ingredient cannabidiol found in the good old-fashioned whiff, which is antipsychotic and protects the brain. The neurochemical changes associated with skunk can permanently damage an immature brain's capacity to remember things. Doctors believe that exposure before the age of fifteen could cause permanent memory loss. And, despite the received street wisdom that cannabis is non-addictive, an increasing number of users develop dependency. Coming off it prompts the common withdrawal symptoms of craving, anxiety, depression and irritability.

True, in the few cases of cannabis-induced psychosis that we treated on Ward 25, any hallucinations were ill-defined and indefinite, delusional beliefs short-lived. Apathy, if anything, seemed to be the defining symptom, and family members reported that such listlessness had been a typical feature of the patient's condition for some time before admission. On the ward these patients were vaguely resentful with a tendency to paranoia and were often incapable of organising themselves for any purpose.

Raymond was one such case. He kept himself very much to himself and, in the opinion of many – patients and staff – was welcome to the lion's share of himself that he kept. When he was out in the ward he was short-tempered and dismissive with everyone. He snapped at Pamela one afternoon when she did not jump to her feet and fetch him the PRN of lorazepam that he demanded.

'I need the fuckin' drugs,' he yelped at her.

'And I'll get them in a minute. I'm dealing with Rosie at the moment.'

'Fuck Rosie! She's always suckin' up to you bastards and gettin' just what she wants.'

'Raymond! I'll be with you in a minute. I'm needed by somebody else right now.'

'Fuck!'

He turned on his heel, to find Gordon and myself at his back.

'Patience, Raymond,' said Gordon. 'Pam's told you that she'll deal with you in a minute.'

'She's always dealin' wi' somebody else!' he snapped and stalked off.

Gordon tutted and followed at a discreet remove, keeping his eye on the irascible Raymond. Theo drew up alongside myself.

'What's all that about, man?'

'Och,' I sighed, 'just Raymondo being his usual good-tempered wee self. He shouldnae smoke dope if it makes him as crabbit as that.'

'Whoah, man, don't be a hypocrite,' said Theo. 'You've had a toke or two in your time. Puff the magic dragon, eh?'

He was right. Back in the day, I had lived in a student flat with a gaggle of other hippies, and not everything that we took into our systems had either been scraped off a frying pan or was strictly legal. There was a certain fragrant substance that we were fond of taking in tufts and rolling in our ciggies or crumbling from cubes into Mary Baker cake mix, when we felt like being a combination of pastry cook and court jester.

But that was a time of youth and excitement. My flatmates and I were high on simply being who we were, set free from the restrictions of home and family for the first time. We always felt that we were set about five seconds ahead of the rest of society. We got the vibe five seconds before anyone else did. We were five seconds quicker on the word on the street and the straws in the wind. We breathed the air five seconds before anyone else did. Oh there were days, certainly, when we indulged in mellow substances; when we fell back on a cloud and watched the vapour trails as everyone else passed by; when we saw their mouths move before we heard what they said, like an out-of-sync soundtrack. And there were times when we lived in days of vibrant colour while everyone else blundered through months of monochrome. These were the days of our lives when the days lived us, rather than the other way round. Although most of the time we were the other way round anyway.

'I know what you're saying, Theo. But the shit we smoked then was completely different from the stuff they smoke today.'

'Dope is dope, man.'

'No. It's not just sticks of tea nowadays. That skunk stuff is up to ten times more powerful than the resin or grass we took. It's been linked to schizophrenia.'

'*Life* is linked to schizophrenia, man.'

'True for you. But it's different stuff, man.'

'I still wouldn't bum anybody else's trip, man.'

'Don't you regret starting drugs, Theo? When you see the way your life has turned out?'

Theo looked at me.

'You can't put a butterfly back in the chrysalis, man,' he said. It might have been one of the most profound things anyone ever said to me.

'That's deep, man,' I told him. 'As deep as anything I ever heard.' He looked pleased.

'When was the first time you toked?' he asked me.

'Hyde Park. London. July' 69.'

'The Stones concert, man?'

'Yep.'

'You ever use a bong, man?'

'A bong? Nah. Hookahs were never our thing.'

'Better for you,' explained Theo. 'The water doesn't just cool the smoke down. It removes some of the tars and carcinogens as well. Try it.'

I promised him I would. I haven't.

Perhaps the most serious case of drug-induced psychosis that I ever witnessed was that of Alasdair. Chemical Allie, as he had been dubbed, had shown no sign of mental illness until well into his twenties, by which time he was married with two young children. According to his notes, he had been a model husband and father, a hard-working breadwinner and payer of the rent until the firm he worked for went bust. He was laid off and could find no other job. Alone in the house, he found that time came in, sat down beside him and wouldn't leave him in peace. He had no hobbies to burn it up; he read no books and gardened no gardens. He and one or two mates took to drugs to annihilate the time. Any drugs. Street drugs or prescription drugs, it didn't matter. They were looking for any kind of portal that would transport them from the ignorant present to a land of canary-yellow skies and sparkling perspectives. Or, failing so, as long as a drug delivered a dunt of any kind, then they would settle for that. Often his mates would arrive at Allie's door with a handful of pills that they had found, or stolen, or been presented with, but which they knew nothing about. Allie would be the guinea pig.

'Go'n try theym, Allie.'

'What are they?'

'Ah donno. They're yella. That's all ah know.'

And Allie would pop one, to see what it was like. His mates would await developments. They watched daytime TV and waited to see what Allie's report was. If he didn't die, then they took the yellow pills too. But one day he took acid and landed himself in the deepest pit of hell. It started with hands reaching out of the walls at him, voices screaming in his head and telling him to kill himself, rats with the faces of humans scurrying around on the floor, and the conviction that he had murdered someone in a gruesome way, butchered the body and forgotten where he had hidden it. When he closed his eyes, he could see terrifying faces hanging in the darkness, faces lit by a strange and lurid light, faces that zoomed around in the space behind his eyelids and ricocheted off his eyeballs with electronic screeching noises. He screamed and hurled himself about the floor, tearing at his eyes in a frantic effort to stop himself from witnessing these horrors. Then he began to feel he was on fire, that tongues of flame were licking at his body. So he *saw* tongues of flame consuming his arms and legs. That was when he burst out of the front door and ran down the street, thumping at his limbs and screaming in abject terror. A classic bad trip.

His bad trip was to go on for years.

In the ward Allie was on constant close obs. He preferred to stay in his room for most of the day, exiting only for a slouch, every two or three hours, to the Smoke Room. Here he ripped through four or five fags one after the other with the suck of a Hoover, before returning to his room. He had a radio on constantly, with the sound turned low, and he lay on his bed with his back to the observer and either slept or tried to. I once asked him how he could bear to have the radio on just as background noise, without being able to distinguish anything said or any music played. I was surprised it didn't drive him up the wall; it certainly did me. I couldn't concentrate on the crossword for it. He looked slightly miffed and said that I shouldn't be doing the crossword; I was supposed to be looking after him. I told him that not every single word that came out of my mouth was to be taken 100 per cent seriously. At which he smiled. Then he said that the background noisery of it was the whole point. The low murmur of the radio kept the voices in his head silent. Or, if it didn't quite manage that, sometimes it could distract him from them enough until they zoomed away again.

He made several attempts on his life and every one of them was serious. I don't mean that it's possible to make a comical one, like trying to die laughing by reading a Conservative manifesto. Simply that each time Allie tried to kill himself, he damn near managed it. And every attempt was bloodier than the previous one.

On one occasion I was on close at his door. He was restless, which made me keep a closer eye on him than usual. Most of the time Allie and I were fairly relaxed with each other. He had never done anything daft on my watch. To this point. Once in a while, for example, he would roll over onto his back and we would have a conversation. Not just about the weather, though, and not about whether Hibs would win the cup this year. He always talked about his illness. How he wanted to shake himself free but could never manage it. How he despaired at the fact that he had not seen his children in years and was afraid he never would again. Whether I thought he could ever be well enough to be free of the Locked Ward and out in the world again. It was during one of these tête-à-têtes that he told me his backstory. I told him that he was showing some progress, however pitifully slight it might be, and that one day he would be out among the real madmen again.

This day, however, he was restless. He turned this way and that in the bed. He shifted his legs. He could not keep still.

'You aw right, Allie?'

'Aye.'

We had this minimalist duologue on a couple of occasions. His answer consisted of a gruff impatient grunt. Something wasn't right with the man. I waited till Luke paced by and attracted his attention before making my disquiet known in dumbshow. I waved to get his eyes on me, then nodded in Allie's direction, wrinkled up my nose, frowned and rocked my hand, extended horizontally, gently from side to side. Finally I made a V with my index and middle fingers, pointed them at my eyes and then pointed at Allie's back. In other words – well, no, in words – I'm not sure about Allie today; we best keep an eye on him. Luke nodded and indicated by describing an ellipse with the point of his right forefinger that he would be in the vicinity. He paced on.

Allie got up.

'Gaun tae the toilet,' he growled.

'Okay.'

The procedure here was straightforward. Everybody is entitled to their privacy. There are times when you step back and let folk do what they have to do, but people who have nonsense in their heads know that this is the procedure. They can often play on our delicacy, using the excuse of the lavatory as an opportunity to do something they shouldn't. It is like the bathroom situation I described earlier. You have to give people the dignity that is everyone's due, but you have to be vigilant as well. Some of these buggers are cuter than Shirley Temple. Bare bum is better than dead body.

Dressed only in trackie bottoms, Allie shuffled to the khazi. I gave him thirty seconds or so.

'You okay, Allie?'

'Aye. Ahm havin' a shit, for fucksake.'

Clever. He knew that that was the answer that would buy him the most time. Nobody wants to keep pestering a man who's having a brown. The next thing might be conversations about texture and consistency, and what was the biggest one you ever did? I gave him another minute. Then I called again.

'You okay, Allie?'

I expected a stinging rejoinder to the effect that he had already told me what was happening. I was prepared for that. Or for another guttural grunt of 'Aye'. But I got nothing. Silence. I was off that chair like – well yes, like shit off a shovel – and tore the lavatory door open.

Allie was seated on the throne all right, but he still had his trackie bottoms on. What he also had was a jagged opening in his neck that was spraying blood all over the wall by the lavvy pan. The little room was like a butcher's counter. Indeed, the gaping wound in his neck reminded me of nothing so much as something you might be served *over* a butcher's counter. I pressed my alarm. The siren started as I roared, 'LUKE! FOR FUCKSAKE!'

Luke came haring in. And in short order so did Gordon and Clyde.

'God Almighty!' said Gordon. It was a God Almighty moment, for sure.

'Get that towel, Dennis,' roared Clyde. 'Pack it into his neck. Stop that bleeding. I'll have to phone the duty doc.'

Luke passed over the bath towel. None too delicately, I compressed the wound. Delicacy was not an option on this occasion. The wound was massive. It needed plenty of pressure. You couldn't have patched it with a

Band-Aid. Meanwhile, Allie just sat there with a slightly bewildered expression on his face, looking from one of us to another.

'How'd he do it?' wondered Gordon.

'CD,' I explained. 'It's still in his hand. Look.'

'Gimme the CD, Allie,' ordered Luke, perfectly prepared if necessary to wrest it from his grip.

It wasn't necessary. Meekly, Allie passed the polycarbonate shard over. It was roughly semicircular in shape with a jagged straight edge. He had obviously broken a disc some time previously and secreted it until such time as he considered he needed to use it. But Allie owned no discs. He listened exclusively to the radio.

'Where'd you get the disc, Allie?' I asked.

'Mary lent it us. I lied an' tellt her I liked Take That an' she lent it us.'

'Fuck, I've no time for Take That either, but I wouldnae snap their discs.'

'Where's the other half?' said Luke.

'Eh?'

'There's two halves tae a disc. Where's the other one? We're no havin' this again.'

'Dinnae ken,' mumped Allie.

'Look for it,' Luke told Gordon.

It wasn't hard to find. It was in Allie's top drawer under a pile of socks.

The duty doc came, told me to take the towel away from Allie's wound and then flinched when he saw the damage done.

'Whew! Plastics will need to see that,' he said.

'Bad as that?' said Allie with some interest.

'Bad as that,' agreed the doctor.

'Aye, you're no gonnae be able to fix that with a darnin' needle,' I joked.

'How's your herringbone stitch?' asked Luke.

'No even wae a Singer sewin' machine,' added Gordon.

Luke and I shook our heads.

Allie got sewn up in Plastic Surgery. If anything, the wound looked crueller when it was stitched. The next time I specialed him, he was back to having a chat with me.

'What made you do that, Allie?' I asked.

'The voices tellt me tae dae it,' he replied.

'Oh, come on,' I said. 'You're a better man than that. If I told you to cut yourself, what would you do?'

'Tell ye tae fuck off,' answered Allie.

'So tell the voices to fuck off,' I said as if I'd just made a major breakthrough in psychiatric methodology.

Allie shook his head pityingly.

'You dinnae understand,' he said. 'You dinnae ken what the voices are like.'

'So tell me.'

'They're as loud as a jet engine sometimes. Maist a the time they just mutter or grumble about how useless ah am. But sometimes they're like the Devil and aw the bad angels an' they're shriekin' in my ears an' they tell me to kill masel. The voices were screamin' at me tae cut masel. Screamin', screamin', screamin'. Loud as a plane. Ah had tae dae it, jist tae make them go away.'

What Allie was describing were command hallucinations, the kind of hallucination in which the patient 'hears' spoken orders from a being within himself, usually to harm himself or other people. I'd read something of them and knew that often the voice or voices seem to the patient to have such absolute control that they have to be obeyed. In many cases the patient feels that the voices are punishing him for some past sin. Sometimes these voices are the voices of loved ones, people from the past or, as in the case of Allie here, the Devil and all his hellish cohorts.

But reading about something is one thing; to hear somebody like Allie describe so vividly what he underwent chilled my blood. I felt such compassion for him. We talk loosely sometimes of everybody having their demons. But it seemed to me that Allie was pursued by a brood of Furies every bit as merciless and unrelenting as those in Greek mythology. Never far from his mind, they sometimes stooped, in as fell a fashion as is imaginable, and sliced to shreds what little remained to him of peace and his own personal identity.

It is possible to have a little insight into this most distressing of conditions. I experienced it during a training course. Try having a normal conversation with someone you know about the most trivial and everyday of subjects. Have them sit facing you. At the same time have one person on one side of you, with their lips close to your ear, singing some little singalong song like 'Bobby Shafto'. Meanwhile, a third person should be at your other ear snarling things like 'You're a fat bastard and you deserve to die; you're a fat bastard and you deserve to die; you're a fat bastard and you deserve to die . . .' You will get some idea of how disturbing it is to try to follow a person's conversation, watching their lips and maybe getting one word in every three, while other voices distract and distress you.

Now imagine that at jet engine volume, commanding you to kill yourself. How do people cope with it? Day in, day out?

'Lord, we know what we are but know not what we may be.'

22

Shut up your doors;
He is attended with a desperate train.
William Shakespeare, *King Lear*

Gordon's sententious remark that life on the ward was like life in the trenches – stretches of boredom punctuated by flashes of violent activity – was beginning to seem well founded. I suppose in every occupation there are routine days, ordinary days, just plain dull days. Despite the fact that I was working in the most interesting job I had known, with some of the most interesting people I ever met, it became true of the Locked Ward too.

There came a time of little change. Days came and then departed, sometimes strings of them. So many of them, in fact, where so little happened that I was forced to examine the days themselves. Often days came that were thin or set at slight angles to the rest of the week. Raw afternoons were not uncommon, nor mornings that were slightly oblong if you looked at them in a certain light. It was not seldom then that I had the unpleasant sensation of somehow unravelling slowly from the spool.

One particular day we were short staffed. We had all grafted in the morning. We had all had shortened morning breaks. We had all done the lunches. And then the afternoon turned out to be sixty-four shades of grey, like a monochrome TV. We were all bored: the patients were bored; the staff were bored. The afternoon, with a slight aftertaste and devoid of any embroidery, sat there like a quite heavy thing and then seeped into evening.

Charlie came to me. Voytek and Bill, who was doing one of his spells in the ward, both wanted an escort to the filling station to buy cigarettes. Also with us for a brief stay at that time was a young man called Gally. Gally was short for Gallagher, but it was the only short thing about him. He was extremely skinny, six feet fourteen and long faced, with extremely jointed limbs. He was a nice guy, but something of a human arthropod. When he was unwell, he had an exaggerated way of walking, which used those arms and legs to astonishing effect, like a caricature of a goose-step performed by the cartoon character Twizzle. He wanted to buy sweets. That made three guys looking for an escort out of the ward.

But, more than that, we also had with us at the time a transsexual from the Borders. He/she didn't stay long with us either, but his/her stay was entirely memorable. I'm not sure at precisely which stage of the transition he/she was. No, I'll stop that. She wanted to be female; she called herself Lola, and she wore female clothes. So it's 'she' and 'her'. I'm not an expert on transgender stuff but it seems to me that transsexuals always wear the most frou-frou and frilly togs that they can get their hands on, almost as if they feel they have to be a caricature of a female to be recognised as one. I hope that's not unfair; I just don't remember seeing any in a plain top and jeans. And, to add a little more pesto to the sauce, Lola wanted a walk too. So then there were four. Four patients all wanting out of the ward and among the Muggles.

Now, strictly speaking, there should have been at least two staff members on that escort, but the ward was busy, it was visiting time and we were short staffed. Charlie asked if I was willing to take them all up to the garage. It would ease the ward situation a fair bit and stop the four craiking on and on about wanting out. I agreed. I told all four to get a coat on; it was bitter cold out there. I would meet them at the airlock door in five minutes. I went for a meditation, put my jacket on, checked my own finances and, having afforded my posse enough time in the green room, met them at the Buffer Zone.

This season Bill was sporting a 1950s swingback swagger faux-ocelot fur coat. He had been seen walking along the street of a local village the previous week in blindingly purple velour trousers and knee-length boots, bare-chested except for a red felt bolero. Coincidentally, he was admitted to us the following day. Green wellingtons set the ocelot off a treat. Lola wore a petal-hem dress in some flimsy material, a sable fur coat and black slingbacks. Her chin was as craggy and blue as Bluto's. Something of a giveaway, I always felt. Voytek was in greatcoat, boots and flying helmet. Gally, thankfully, was quite soberly dressed in a denim jacket and jeans. You couldn't call him unobtrusive, though. It was not an unobtrusive group of people. They were about as unobtrusive as pantomime horses.

And so into the airlock and then out into the hospital we went. By the time we reached the ground floor, I realised that this was maybe not such a good idea. It was evening visiting time. There were people everywhere, in lifts, wards and corridors: old people, middle-aged people and young people; teenagers and children; sad people, worried people and jolly people; porters, nurses, doctors, technicians and tradesmen.

Out of the lift we tumbled and along the main corridor we progressed. Gally was in front, striding out, swinging his extendable arms and kicking his extendable legs. Bill loped along behind him in his ocelot swagger, grinning like a turnip lantern, chattering to every passer-by. Lola tripped along next to him on her ludicrous heels, her big stubbly jaw jutting out over her sable coat. And I brought up the rear with Biggles.

People were running away. Jumping into cupboards. Diving behind trolleys. Scrambling into bins and pulling the lid on after them.

All that was missing was a stirring rendition of 'Entry of the Gladiators', a strongman carrying a barbell, somebody dressed as Uncle Sam on stilts and an oiled Levantine breathing fire to make the circus complete. It was one of my favourite moments in all my seven and a half years in the Locked Ward. In fact, few moments in my entire life come close to it. I've never been prouder to be in a company.

And then we passed through the big front doors of the hospital and out into the night, where we turned into winking golden fireflies and vanished in the darkness.

23

. . . they shall yet belie thy happy years,
That say thou art a man; Diana's lip
Is not more smooth and rubious; thy small pipe
Is as the maiden's organ, shrill and sound,
And all is semblative a woman's part.

William Shakespeare, *Twelfth Night*

Anent the person Lola, Gordon had a comment or two to make. We had expected it. It came around the breakfast table the morning after Lola had returned – or rather, had *been* returned, like a parcel – to the Borders. She had been with us a week. The conversation experienced a momentary lull, and that gave Gordon his chance.

'You know that bloke, Lola?'

'What about her?' growled Charlie.

'Well!' said Gordon, as if that was enough said.

'Well what?'

'Well, what's *that* all aboot, eh?'

'How d'you mean, Gordon?' said Pamela.

'Well. A bloke wantin' to be a wumman. 'S no right, is it? If you're a bloke, you're a bloke. Surely.'

'And if you're a boke, you're a boke,' said Rona pointedly.

'You know anything about transgenderism?' asked Charlie.

'Evidently not,' said Pamela. 'Look, some people believe they were born into the wrong body. Not just believe it,' she added quickly, 'actually *feel* it in every cell of their body.

That they're the wrong gender. That they should be male instead of female, or female instead of male.'

'How can you be born in the wrong body?' persisted Gordon. 'I mean, it's no as if there's a choice in the womb, an' the wean picks a male body instead of a female one, is it?'

'It's complicated,' said Pamela. 'But, basically, what happens is that when a baby's born they're assigned a sex – male or female – on the evidence of their genitalia. Okay? Vulva – wee girl; penis – wee boy. It's the traditional way. But some folk grow up feeling that this is either a false identity or sometimes not a complete one.'

'If you've got a cock you're a boy; if it's a fanny you're a girl. That's what makes folk what they are. You dinnae get a leopard thinkin' it should really have been a tiger, dae ye? It's got spots, it's a leopard. Disnae matter if it *feels* it should hae stripes. Or tries tae join its spots up *intae* stripes. Or says that it feels like a tiger in a leopard's fur. Dis it? It's still a leopard.'

'What's your point, caller?' growled Charlie.

'It's the same wi' folk. Disnae matter if they *think* they're female, or if their hale body *feels* it's female. If they've got a bobby, they're a bloke. A fuckin' mixed-up bloke maybe. But a bloke just the same.'

There was a brief pause.

'You don't have a lot of humanity or sympathy for these people, do you?' said Pamela.

'How no?'

'Some of them are extremely unhappy about their condition. They're confused and feel trapped. They are often laughed at and bullied. Some of them develop mental illnesses as a result. Some get suicidal. We're here to help people who have these feelings. Not to sneer at them.'

'Who's sneerin'?' Gordon almost screamed. 'I'm no sneerin'; I'm just sayin' . . . well you said it for me. When you sayed they develop mental illness. Mah point is that surely thinkin' you're a woman when you're a bloke *is* a mental illness. If somebody thinks they're Napoleon or Jesus or John Lennon, Dr Bankstreet says that's a symptom ae a mental illness and she brings them in here an' treats them till they get better. So, if that bloke, whatever his name was . . .'

'Lola.'

'. . . his real name, whatever his real name was, calls hisself Lola, dresses up in a tutu and high heels, but still has a chin like Desp'rate Dan, an' still has his meat an' two veg intact, surely that's a symptom ae a mental illness just the same?'

'It's much more than that,' said Charlie shortly. 'That's too reductive. Your analogy's all to fuck.'

'I'm suspicious of anybody,' said Pamela, 'who's so dead keen on conformity. Why should everybody be the same?'

'All I'm sayin',' said Gordon, 'is that surely it's obvious when a wean's got boys' bits or girls' bits.'

'Not always,' said Pamela. 'Genitals don't come in identical editions. No two penises are alike; no two vulvas are alike. Sometimes it's hard to differentiate.'

'Why is it always you that ends up talking like that?' asked John, finishing his porridge. 'It upsets me. I'm at a bad age.'

Pamela laughed. Charlie cut a chunk of sausage and dipped it in his egg. Gordon sat silently for a moment. Then he spoke again.

'Okay,' he said. 'New thing.'

'Okay,' said Charlie. 'Shoot.'

'See Lola, right?'

'New thing? Same thing,' said Luke.

'Naw. Wait a minute. See Lola. He wants tae be a lassie. So why does he no get the hormones an' get his thingmae taken aff?'

'New thing, right enough,' said Luke.

'Because,' said Charlie, with infinite patience, 'the hormone treatment that she would need would be bad grammar wi' the psychotropic medication that she's on and they have to see that she's well enough to come off the meds before they can even try it.'

'Has to be clear for – what is it, Charlie? – three months?'

'Somethin' like that, Pam.'

'Aw, right.'

Gordon sat quietly and spooned his Rice Krispies into his mouth for a while.

'Talkin' about sexual confusion,' said Luke, 'how's the Widow Twankey?'

Gordon was enamoured of an older woman in his native village. She was a lady in her late forties, a widowed schoolteacher with a grown-up son two years older than Gordon. That she was older, glamorous and sophisticated where he was callow and rough as a badger's arse fazed him not a jot. The poor fool doted on her. He smouldered like a briquette with unrequited love. He had been foolhardy enough to mention his feelings one day and had been mercilessly ragged ever since. Over many conversations around the meal table we had elicited the following information: that she was tall with a good figure; that her hair was collar-length and dark, starting to grey slightly; that she drove a dark blue Merc; that she taught maths at a high school in the city and her name was Imogen.

'Imogen!' snorted Luke. 'Must be middle class wi' a name like that. Oot ae your league, farm boy.'

'She's posh, aye, if that's what you mean,' said Gordon.

'Does she speak proper?'

'Oh aye, right posh.'

'Imogen? That's a name fae classical literature, intit, Dennis?' said Luke.

'Not sure about classical literature, but it's from Shakespeare. Imogen is a character in *Cymbeline*. She dresses up as a man at one point.'

'Ho, kinky!' John laughed. 'That the attraction, Gordy boy? That explains the interest in Lola!'

Gordon looked miserable.

'You don't seem to be getting much joy from being in love with her,' I said.

'Well, she disnae ken how ah feel. An' she's no likely tae feel the same, is she?'

'She got a man?' asked Clyde. 'No point in getting your kecks kinked over a woman if she got somebody already.'

'Naw,' said Gordon. 'She just goes tae her work in the mornin', and comes hame at half five. That's it. Marks jotters. Does the gardenin'.'

'You seem to know a lot about her,' said Rona.

'Stalker,' said John shortly. 'Follows her about the village. Spies on her.'

'You better watch youself, man,' said Clyde. 'End up with your name on a register somewhere.'

'Ah'm no a stalker,' said Gordon indignantly. 'I just see her about the place.'

'Does she know you?' asked Rona.

'Oh aye. She knows who I am. Says hello if we meet. She knows my mother through the Rural.'

'The Rural?' said Rona. 'That's a good sign.'

'How?'

'Means she's looking for something to fill up her spare time.'

'So?'

'So she's no got a *man*. Or he would be filling it up.'

'Smart boy wanted,' I said.

'Oh, she wouldnae look at *me*,' said Gordon modestly. 'She's far too sophisticatit for me.'

'Talk to her,' said Rona. 'You cannae get to know her if you don't talk to her.'

'What'll I say?' asked Gordon.

'Hi, Imogen. You up for a night bitin' the pilla?' suggested John.

'John!' Rona checked him like a schoolmarm herself.

'Aye, very good,' mumped Gordon.

'Don't plan anything,' said Rona. 'Just talk to her naturally. About whatever seems right. Get to know her. This is a person we're talking about. Not just a chance of a . . . a quickie.'

'A quickie, Rona!' said John. 'First Pamela, now *you're* at it. I'll need to go and lie down in a darkened room.'

Gordon thought for a second.

'I was thinkin' of goin' tae the church she goes tae. Maybe meet her there.'

'Good idea,' said Rona. 'You know what church she goes to?'

'Oh aye. The EU church.'

'Evangelicals?' said Luke. 'She'll be too holy-holy for any nonsense wi' the likes of you, Gordy boy.'

'Naw, naw,' said Rona. 'The EU church isnae the Wee Frees. They're quite relaxed about things. They say it's up to the individual to accept God. Something like that.'

'Oh well. You're quids in, son,' said John.

Gordon may have gone to the EU church and may even have seen Imogen there. But he never spoke his love. Nor got her to love him back. Not as far as I know. I'm sure we'd have heard of it if he had. He just went on, day to day and month to month, silently worshipping at his middle-class, tall and well-figured shrine. His looks of longing in her direction probably burned smoking, jasmine-scented tracks in the air. But no joy. The religion didn't seem to do much for his equanimity either.

24

Away! the foul fiend follows me!
Through the sharp hawthorn blows the cold wind
William Shakespeare, *King Lear*

Oh, and talking about religion . . . The hospital had a
chaplaincy. Most do, although our lot preferred to big
themselves up by calling themselves the Department of
Spiritual Welfare. Forgive me for sounding cynical, but
almost any venue could do the same. My local certainly
fulfils that function for many. But it sounds quasi-medical
enough for a hospital. I don't doubt they do a lot of good. I
doubt everything they believe in, but I don't doubt they mean
well and that they lighten the burden for some. I suppose a
shoulder to cry on's a shoulder to cry on, secular or religious.

The Department of Spiritual Welfare had five regulars
in the squad, two women and three men, plus a flying picket
or two of ministers, priests and nuns who visited wards as
part of their pastoral duties, laying on hands and telling the
sick to take up their beds and walk. (I know; I can't help it.
I caught flippancy at an early age and it went straight to the
brain. I've never been able to shift it. If the hospital had
had the atheist equivalent of a chaplaincy – I don't know;
a Department of Rational Welfare, say – I'd be taking the
piss out of that too. Sneering at the idea that life is defined
by its end. All very well until you're near it.) Anyhow, I
have no objection to anyone troubling deaf heaven with

208

their bootless cries. Especially if it helps them feel a wee bit better. Just so long as they realise that talking to a doctor probably does more good. But I ramble.

Each ward had a cleric from the D of SW assigned to it, and the Locked Ward's padre was a slightly built man called Nicol. Despite being happily married and having begat a sizeable brood of Nicolettes (these Holy Joes certainly like the old hochmagandy), he was as camp as light opera. He was also as savage as a wolverine when it came to discussing God and related mystical matters.

I've never liked Nicol as a first name. It's always seemed to me to be one of those reversible names like Grant Crawford/Crawford Grant or Finlay Ross/Ross Finlay. And Nicol's full name might even have been Nicol McNicol, which is even sillier. But I could be making that up. Silly names are among the many bees that buzz around in my big bonnet. Jesse Boot. Ford Madox Ford. The Reverend Canaan Banana. Isambard Kingdom Brunel. Nicol McNicol. But there I am, all over the map again.

At least once a week Nicol would arrive on the ward, trailing slightly perfumed clouds of glory, and spend some time talking and listening to some of the sickest patients.

I admired Nicol for doing what he did. Many of the patients cared no more for religion than I did but were much more direct about their wish for him to leave them alone. What I didn't like about him is something I dislike about many God botherers – most of them, in fact. And that is their absolute certainty of the truth of their particular brand of gibberish and their searing contempt – far worse than any atheist's – for the gibberish of any other religion. Only they know the layout of the Happy Hunting Grounds, and only they know where to find the rope ladder to get up there.

Nicol was like that. He pretended to have respect for any form of belief, but he only respected his own. Judaism, Islam and Hinduism he saw as exotic delusions. Any other sect of Christianity, especially Catholicism, he saw as a cadre of misbelievers. Laughable, really, if it didn't regularly have tragic consequences in the world at large.

Occasionally, after he had seen the patients, he would consent to stop and have a coffee. I used to like breaking a lance with him at times like these.

'Do you really believe God exists?' I'd asked him one time.

'Believe? No. I *know* God exists.'

'You *know* it? You've seen him, spoken to him, have you?'

'No, but he has spoken to me.'

'Yeah? I think you'll find he's spoken to 75 per cent of the patients we get in here.'

'Cheap point.'

'Cheap argument. You've given no evidence for God existing.'

'Look around you. The world. The sky. The mountains. The seas. The stars. How do you think they got there?'

'They're just aspects of one lump of rock among millions. How they got here . . . science can answer that better than me. I'm a humble English graduate.'

'Science!' Nicol snorted. 'Science doesn't know everything. It can't explain everything.'

'No, not yet. But it admits that it can't. Yet. Some day it will. What's your alternative? Magic? Abracadabra? No, I'm not swallowing that.'

'Some day you'll see the light.'

'Maybe. If I do, I hope it's your bonfire, you smug shit.'

'Lord forgive him for he knows not what he does.'

And so on.

He was sitting with Clyde and Luke at a table in the Dayroom one afternoon when I sauntered in.

'Aha,' I said by way of greeting. 'Let us alone, what have we to do with thee, Jesus of Nazareth?'

Luke and Clyde looked at me and then looked at each other with that 'Here he goes again' look. Nicol just gave me a tolerant smile.

'You know,' he said, 'for a heathen, you know a fair bit of Scripture.'

'Know it better than some of the whited sepulchres that pitch up at church and chapel of a weekend, that's for sure.'

'You know what they say: the Devil can quote Scripture for his own ends.'

'Know it better than you, you bloody old Pharisee. It's from *The Merchant of Venice*. And it actually says, "The Devil can cite Scripture for his purpose." So there.'

'You know, I can't imagine how a man can live a life of purpose, a meaningful life, without God,' he said.

'That's because you're conditioned to think that way. Go on, throw that Bible away. Free yourself. Live a bit.'

'And then die and spend eternity without God? I don't think so.'

'We're all going to do that,' I said. 'Spend eternity without God. And without Santa Claus. And without the Tooth Fairy.'

'What I don't understand,' said Nicol, 'is if you don't believe in God, heaven and hell . . .'

'Which I don't.'

' . . . what makes you live a good life? That's assuming that you do, of course. Assuming that your only real sin is intellectual arrogance.'

'That's an old one,' I said. 'I do try to live a good life. Do the right things. But I don't refrain from murder or rape or theft because I'm scared of going to hell if I do these things. I just don't do them because they're bad things to do to people. Like I try to help people in life because it's the right thing to do. Not because some old pooperoo with a white beard and a Wee Willie Winkie nightdress will take me into heaven.'

'Who's the old man in the white beard and gown?' snorted Nicol contemptuously. 'Nobody thinks of God in that anthropomorphic way nowadays.'

'I meant the Maharishi,' I said.

Nicol smiled.

'Bloody old hippy,' laughed Clyde, who was a believer himself, I think.

'We must disagree, I fear,' said Nicol.

'At least you pay me the intellectual compliment of not trying to convert me,' I said.

'Easier to convert horsepower to BTU,' said Luke.

'Somebody once said,' said Nicol, 'that once a man stops believing in God, the problem is not that he believes in nothing, but that he will believe in anything.'

'I think it was Chesterton,' I said. 'But what about Muslims who believe in God, but call him Allah? Or Jews who believe in God but call him Yahweh? Will they go to heaven too? Or are they as deluded as I am?'

'God says the righteous will sit by his right hand on the Day of Judgement. Righteous Jews and Muslims will be there.'

'And me?'

'Your arse will fry,' he said with a guffaw.

It was the week after that little conversation that Charlie phoned off sick. Geraldine took over the running of the ward in his absence. Like Charlie, she would not be fucked about by those higher up the line, and she demanded that, the ward being as it then was, we get a male replacement for Charlie. She got one.

His first name was Jacob, and his second was one of those long, melodious and evocative African surnames. Jacob was in his fifties, small, stout and balding. His skin was as black as two o'clock in the morning and his accent was beautifully rich and African. Geraldine brought him up the ward to introduce him to the rest of us. I was seated at the Station with John and Luke, having a smoke.

'Boys, this is Jacob,' said Geraldine.

'Hi, Jacob.'

'These guys will keep you right,' said Geraldine and went.

Jacob extended his hand to John.

'Hallo, I'm Jacob.'

'I'm John.'

'Pleased to meet you, John.'

'I'm Luke.'

'Pleased to meet you, Luke.'

'I'm Dennis.'

He stopped and looked at me as if I'd said something silly. Then he smiled indulgently at me.

'Are you sure you don't mean Daniel?'

'No. Dennis.'

'Are you sure? Not Daniel?'

'Fairly sure. I've been carrying it around with me for fifty years.'

'Not Daniel?'

'Why the hell would it be Daniel?'

'Dennis is not biblical.'

The other two pissed themselves quietly in the background.

'Naw,' said I, 'and neither am I. Don't give me any of that biblical codswallop. I'm only sorry my name isn't Darwin.'

That kind of blind unctuous religiosity really grates on my nerves. I'm sure Jacob was a decent man but his sanctimony would have been a severe impediment to our friendship. The possibility never arose.

It was at this point that Stannie emerged from his room and came wandering down the corridor towards us.

'Stannie,' said John.

'Gentlemen,' said Stannie.

Then he did a superbly executed double-take, stopped abruptly and stared at Jacob.

'Are you . . . *Clyde*?' he asked as if stupefied.

Now I think I made Jacob's physical description clear. Apart from the fact that his skin tone was four or five shades darker than Clyde's, he was twenty-five years older, a foot and a half shorter, five stones heavier and a fair degree balder. How could this have been Clyde, unless he had seriously pissed off a witch?

Nor was Stannie a halfwit or an uncultured boorish man. Jacob was not the first black man he had seen. Nor even the second. Quite why he thought that this older, smaller and fatter man was Clyde is still beyond me. Even given the fact that Clyde was the only non-Caucasian member of staff he had encountered in this narrow context, it still required a fair sag of the imagination to take one for the other.

But any conjecture at the time was rapidly terminated by a piercing scream from Ursula, closely followed by the shrill of the alarm. I glanced at the board.

'Allie's room!'

And there we pelted. Ursula was standing at the opened door, the chair she had been sitting in kicked back. She was shrinking from the sight in the room. I got to the door first and looked in as John and Luke thundered up behind me.

Allie was sitting in his chair, naked to the waist. His arms were held rigidly by his sides, and he was twisting his hands around as if in extreme pain. His eyes had rolled back in his head so that all we could see were the yellowish whites. His lips were filmed with a slime of greyish mucus. He was rolling his head repeatedly around on his neck, clockwise, clockwise, always clockwise. His features contorted themselves into various terrifying expressions of agony. And from his scummed mouth emanated a low bestial sound: a grumbling, rasping snarl like some wild animal that's been disturbed.

'He just started doin' this!' screamed Ursula.

'Fucksake!' said John. 'What the fuck is wrong with him?'

'He is possessed!' hissed a horrified Jacob, who had appeared behind John and Luke.

Certainly, if ever a human being looked like he was possessed by a devil, an unclean spirit, poor Allie did at that moment. Now his voice rose to a querulous growl.

'Fuck!' said John.

'What the fuck is wrong wi' this man?'

'Withdrawal,' snapped Geraldine, appearing at the door beside us. 'He's been palming his meds. He needs to be sedated right away. Ursula, phone the duty doc. You guys stay here till I draw something up. Jacob, can you do the coffees and things? Here's the kitchen key.'

John, Luke and I stayed put while the others bustled off. We watched Allie in horror. Clockwork robotic movements.

No eyes. Mouth seeping pus or whatever. Grinding his teeth. And that animalistic growl.

'Fuck,' I said. 'I don't believe all that demonic possession shit, but this would be enough to convince anybody.'

'Terrifyin',' agreed Luke.

'You guys ever seen anything like this?' I asked.

'Never,' said Luke.

'Never as bad, anyway,' said John.

'Poor fucker,' said Luke. 'He must be in torments.'

And then Allie lunged off the chair towards us, snarling and spitting, lashing out. It was as if Luke's words had angered the beast within. Only there wasn't a beast within. He was just extremely ill. It was easy to see, however, why people in biblical times, with no knowledge of medicine or mental illness, would think that some malignant spirit had taken possession of someone. Especially showing the symptoms Allie was showing.

He flattened John against the lavatory door and grabbed his neck, compressing it while he growled and talked Demon. Luke grabbed him by the shoulder and pulled him back, easing his grip on John's neck. John squeezed his hand under one of Allie's to alleviate the pressure. I took hold of Allie's right hand, pulling his thumb back. (It's always easier to detach the thumb than the fingers; there are four fingers and only one thumb.) Suddenly Allie's grip loosened, and he fell back on Luke, dragging me with them. On the bed Luke slid from under him as John and I grabbed him from the top and put him into the restraint position. It took all our combined strength to keep him there; he was struggling and bucking around like a bull. Geraldine came back with the jag.

'Gonnae need the rhino gun, I think, Gerry,' said John.

'God! What happened to your neck, John?' It was very red and showed quite clearly Allie's fingermarks.

'Oh, your man here decided to give me a wee cuddle,' said John.

'I'll look at that in a minute,' said Geraldine. 'You'll need to hold him still.'

'We're tryin',' said Luke.

'Duty doc's on his way,' said Ursula, suddenly there.

'Get some guys from 24,' called Geraldine. 'We need to keep Allie still to jag him.'

Ursula took off again. Allie continued to rock and roll, growl and snarl. His eyes, which had been back to facing the right way while he attacked John, were rolling back into his head again. Two male nurses from Ward 24 joined us. It took the five of us to hold Allie still enough for Geraldine to jag him. He subsided after ten minutes. And then he needed another two jags in the next couple of hours before he got back to the way he had been.

The duty doc confirmed Geraldine's diagnosis. Allie had been spitting out his meds for a day or two without anyone noticing. He had been an excellent complier up to that point. Some antipsychotics are so powerful that sudden withdrawal from them can have the most drastic effects. Nausea, diarrhoea, dizziness, tremors and marked psychotic symptoms are among the most regularly encountered ones. Nobody had seen an effect quite like Allie's before. Geraldine was a skilled nurse; she knew immediately what the problem was. People like her are invaluable on a ward like 25.

Allie got better in a day or two. He was profusely apologetic to John, who shrugged his apologies off with a wry smile.

'All part of the rich tapestry, Allie, pal.'

We never saw Jacob again. I wasn't sorry. I'm sure he was a reasonable guy and a good enough nurse. I just didn't fancy having to apologise all the time for not being called Nicodemus.

25

A robin red breast in a cage
Puts all Heaven in a rage.
William Blake, 'Auguries of Innocence'

Two or three years into my spell on the ward, Charlie made an executive decision to keep the bedded area open at all times, unless there was a specific reason for closing it, such as an organised search for drugs or weapons. He consulted Dr Bankstreet and the Mental Welfare Commission, and then told the domestic staff that the area was to stay open all day and all of the night. Which might have given Ray Davies an idea for a song.

The problem had been that under the earlier system, once patients had been roused from their slumbers and ushered through to break their collective fasts, the area had been locked until two o'clock. This was to allow the domestics to clean the area undisturbed. Unfortunately, one effect of having twelve very ill patients comparatively restricted in their movements was sometimes to cause confrontations and even fights. Other than the Smoke Room, there was really only the Dayroom for them to congregate in. Some patients used the GP Room at certain times, but mostly they lounged about the Dayroom, watching TV, or paced the corridors. It was inevitable that occasional disgreements would arise, and that these disagreements would sometimes turn violent.

It was usually over nothing of any importance. One patient attempting to enter the Dayroom while another was exiting might bump shoulders and bang! They were off.

'Watch it, bastard!'

'Who you calling a bastard? I'll fucking flatten you.'

'Oh aye? I'll rip your nose aff an' pish in the hole.'

Whoosh! Fight, fight!

A lot of the squaring-up and shouting amounted to little more than chest beating. Most of the fights were no more than spats, like two hares kick-boxing in a field. Quickly over. But sometimes, depending on the patients, fights were hard and raised blood. We had to separate the antagonists and calm them down, keep them separate, usher one to the Smoke Room or out into the courtyard while the other stayed in the Dayroom, give their tempers time to abate. But resentments often simmered away. And there was very little space for rivals to keep out of each other's way.

Opening up the bedded area solved that problem at a stroke. After breakfast patients were free to go back to their own rooms and chill, if they wished. Many did. Some lay on their beds and slept; some listened to music. Some read. One or two had portable TVs brought in by visitors. Patients were encouraged to make their own beds and be responsible for their own laundry, and many passed their time in these day-to-day activities. And there was still the Smoke Room and the Dayroom if they felt like socialising. (It meant an end to staff meals taken together, though. Too many areas where trouble might flare up. We took our meals in twos.)

To be sure, many patients paced the corridors. Back and forth, from the rooms to the front door, up to the Dayroom and thence to the rooms, back and forth. Back and forth, back and forth. One or two did it for exercise, to keep themselves active. But some did it repetitively, compulsively. They felt caged. And they were, mentally and physically. Imprisoned. Locked up. Removing a person's freedom, no matter how necessary it is deemed, or how well intentioned, is a serious thing to do, with potentially far-reaching consequences. Most of the patients were detained against their will, sectioned under the Mental Health Act, so it was no surprise that they looked on the ward as a prison and the staff as warders.

It is also a controversial thing to do. It is done by medical professionals to ensure the safety of the patient and of others. There is a school of thought, though, which maintains that to lock a patient up increases the likelihood of aggression. There is evidence that patients feel that they are just prisoners under another name. They become depersonalised and stigmatised. Not to mention resentful, surly and mutinous. This makes violent incidents, including assaults on staff, more likely. They are also more likely to self-harm and refuse meds if they are locked up. And the increase in suicidal ideation within the ward rises significantly. Research shows that about 150 patients succeed in committing suicide in locked wards in the UK each year, despite the locks and the increased security. Some argue that wards should not be locked but that staff should monitor the doors to check who enters and leaves.

There is no doubt that the locked ward has a custodial feel to it. Some professionals think it is precisely the opposite of therapeutic, as a result of this. But there are persuasive counter-arguments. The locked door does provide staff with a degree of control over patients, seen as essential until the patient recovers. Much as they may dislike it, the locked door does provide patients with a sense of security and safety, and even protection in some cases. Some patients – not many, but some – feel that the locked ward is a place where the world cannot harm them.

There are, indeed, many negative aspects to locking patients up. The only comment I would make, having worked in 25 for many years, is that to open up this kind of ward would require a much greater staff-to-patient ratio. And that's not going to happen in the current economic climate, no matter how therapeutic it might be. And there would still be patients who, for any of several reasons, would require to be locked up.

Still, I could not help but feel sorry for the patients, as they padded the floors of the ward restlessly, endlessly, trying to kill time or distract themselves from unwelcome thoughts and feelings. Sometimes I'd come upon a patient standing by a window, wistfully gazing out at the hospital grounds. The big outdoors. There was never anything exciting going on out there, but that was not the point. The point was that it *was* out there; the patients were not.

One night a young woman called Frances was sitting by the Dayroom window, her chin in her hand, looking out at the darkness and the cold moon, saying nothing, doing nothing, just looking like she was waiting for the return of Ulysses.

'All right, Frances? Bored?'

'No. Just wondering when I'll get out of here.'

'Won't be long now. You're doing well.'

'Yeah? Nice to hear that. Except it's not you that makes that decision. It's Dr Bankstreet. She's a lot less likely than you to let me go soon.'

'Oh, I don't know.'

'Do you know how many months I've spent in this ward and wards like it?'

'No.'

'No. I don't either, but it's months and months. Years of my life, probably. I wonder how many of those months I could have been outside. Living. You know – living? Nothing big or important. Just doing the shopping, hanging out the washing, talking to people. Eating meals when I want, not when somebody tells me to. Going out the door when I felt like it. The sort of thing you do all the time.'

'Jeez, Frances, when you say it like that . . .'

'Yeah.'

'You must have needed to be in, though.'

'Oh aye. Some of the time I've been really unwell, I know that. But the doctors keep you in longer than they need to. And there's an awful lot of really unwell people out there, anyway. I wonder how much Dr Bankstreet would like it if somebody took *her* liberty away when she didn't feel well. Because they were an expert.'

26

Merely innocent flirtation,
Not quite adultery, but adulteration.
Lord Byron, *Don Juan*

The hounds of spring were on winter's traces. The grass was growing green everywhere; buds were budding; birds were warbling; hares were acting daft in meadow and lea. Spring is when a young man's fancy lightly turns to thoughts of love. Spring, sweet spring, is the year's something king, after all; the only pretty ring time, hey ding-a-ding and all that. And one particular young man was admitted at this appropriate time. With a hey and a ho and a hey nonny-no. Although I think Edward's fancy lightly turned to thoughts of love no matter what the time of year.

He was admitted from a hospital in the city. A thoroughly engaging character with a broad smile, he was popular with just about everyone – staff, fellow patients, medical team, domestics, porters, visitors, several people in the hospital shop, children, dogs and most of the inhabitants of Tristan da Cunha. He suffered from a bipolar condition.

The basic thing about bipolar illness is easy to remember – mood swings. Periods of depression then periods of elevation. Or mania. Edward seemed to me to be almost permanently in a state of euphoria. He was sunnily disposed towards everybody and constantly excited about every little aspect of his day. Twenty times a day I passed him in the corridor, and every single time this conversation, or something very like it, took place.

'Dennis! Dennis! Hi, Dennis. How you doin'?'

'I'm fine, Edward. How are you?'

'In the pink, Dennis. In the pink. Top of the world. Have to go. Things to do, folk to see. Cheerio, Dennis.'

'Toodloo, Edward.'

He had the most grandiose notions. He had a hundred ideas a day: setting up a recording studio in the city and making his fortune by discovering the new Beatles; writing a graphic novel about a superhero who wins back independence for Scotland; discovering a cure for cancer; anything.

A typical example.

'Hi, Dennis, hi. How you doin'?'

'I'm fine, Edward. How are you?'

'In the pink, Dennis, in the pink. You ever been to Australia, Dennis?'

'No, never.'

'I'm goin'. Goin' to Australia when I get out of here. Goin' backpackin'. Australia, aye. Canberra. Sydney Opera House. You can fly to Australia in twenty-four hours. Have to stop off in places, like. Cannae fly the whole way in a oner. Singapore. Aye, I'm goin' to Australia.'

'Got any relatives in Australia, Edward?'

'Relatives? Naw. No problem. Backpackin'. Stay in hostels and that. Cheap way of doin' it. Easy.'

'Why Australia?'

'Down under. Ayers Rock. The natives call it Uluru. Have to see that before I die. Mystical qualities.'

Theo was passing at this point, on his way to the Smoke Room.

'Uluru, man? Yeah. Far out. Sacred to the aborigines, man. Don't take anything from it, though. Like a rock or a plant or any shit like that. You'll end up cursed.'

'Oh no, no, I wouldn't. Nothing like that. Just to see it.'

Satisfied, Theo moved on.

'Takes quite a bit of money to fly to Australia, I would think,' I said.

'Yeah, I'll sell off a few of my investments.'

This was another of Edward's grandiose ideas – that he was a wheeler-dealer in the financial world. He was always asking for permission to use the phone to contact his people in the City. He carried a small notebook at all times, in which he had, as far as I could see, nothing but columns and columns of figures, separated by mathematical symbols and underlined in random places with heavy scores. The secret of his success.

'Any chance of using the phone, Dennis?'

'Sure.'

While I was fishing my keys out of my pocket and unlocking the Phone Room door, he explained his latest wheeze.

'Just arranging a loan with the bank. There's a very nice detached villa in the property section today. Going for a song. A snip. Get that, fix it up, sell it on. One two three. Easy as winkie. Thanks, Dennis.'

And in he would scuttle to the phone with his scheme to become the new Gulbenkian. I never heard any more about the property or the proposed jaunt to Oz. But that was always the way of things with Edward. He was always excited to the point of bursting about his projects at the time, but they were dropped quietly and quickly when a new one took their place.

He would stride down the ward, singing. He was especially fond of heavy metal music and would carol suddenly as anybody passed him. 'The ice of spides; the ice of spides' was a particular favourite. He had been the drummer in a band at one time.

Edward did a fair bit of walking too. His chosen ground was the courtyard. He asked Charlie how many times round would constitute a mile. Charlie reckoned maybe ten, but he couldn't be sure. Might have been twenty. And Edward would spend half an hour a day walking speedily round the courtyard, following the lines of the walls, with that slightly hyper-looking heel-and-toe walk of Olympic race walkers. Then he'd burst into the ward, flushed and puffing.

'Ten miles. Ten miles, Dennis. Just walked ten miles. Fucked now. Off to bed.'

And off he would stride to lie down on top of his bed. But he'd be back on the floor ten minutes later, with a new idea and telling everybody that he was in the pink. It was impossible not to like the guy.

The other thing about Edward was that he was perhaps the most sexual person I've ever met. He was always on about sex, the girls he'd slept with and the things they'd done when he did. I used to tell him it was private business and that I didn't want to hear anything about it. He'd stop, say, 'Oh. Right. Sorry, Dennis. Nae harm done,' and walk away. But an hour later he'd be back, telling me and Luke about the night he'd flattened a field of corn with a married woman from Ashby de la Zouch.

'She was up here on holiday, like. Nice woman. And up for it, nae messin'. Met her at the working men's club. She was with a pal. Me and my mate split them on the dance floor and then her and me headed off to do the business, you know . . .'

'Edward!'

'Sorry, boys. All boys together, you know? You've been there. You've done it tae. Anyway. Nae harm done. You couldnae let me into the Phone Room, Luke, could you? Cheers. Appreciate it.'

He also had the biggest penis that any of us had ever seen on a human being. And, like most guys who are gifted in the trouser department, had no problem about showing it to anybody and everybody at the slightest opportunity. The first time it happened to me, I was doing the breakfast round, knocking on doors and calling on all who were eager to partake of hospital porridge or soggy cereal. I knocked on Edward's door and opened it. He came out of his lavatory, dressed only in a pair of shorts.

'That's the breakfast in, Ed, old son.'

'Right, Dennis. Be right there. Right there. Dennis, would you do me a favour?'

'What is it?'

'Would you take a look at my penis for me?'

'Rather not, Edward. I'll be honest with you.'

'I'd like you to look at it.'

'I've seen penises before, Ed.'

'Aye, I know, I know, I don't mean that. I don't mean anything, you know . . . I mean, tell me what's wrong with it.'

'What *is* wrong with it?'

'I don't know.'

And, on the word, he slipped his boxers down his thighs and there was the organ in question. It was impressive, I have to say.

'Should it be *like* that?' he asked.

Resisting the temptation to crack the obvious joke that I wished mine was like that, I said rather, 'Like what?'

'Well . . . the rash. The red rash.'

'I don't see a red rash.'

'Look closer.'

'I'm looking close enough,' I said. 'There's nothing wrong with it. Put it away.'

'If you say so.'

'I do. Now, breakfast.'

Without a murmur of protest, Edward pulled up his boxers and got dressed, then emerged for breakfast.

I was not alone in being vouchsafed a keek at Edward's genitalia. Most of the guys went through the same routine at one time or another in the first few weeks of his stay. The rash worried him. And then Pamela got the big invitation. I was having a drag in the Smoke Room with a few patients when she stuck her head round the door.

'Dennis, have you got a minute?'

Fortunately, at that precise time I had several. I nipped my weed and followed her out the door.

'Will you come with me up to Edward's room?'

'Sure. Why?'

'He wants me to have a look at his penis.'

'Your turn, is it? Thought he'd get round to the girls eventually.'

'I'm not laughing. He says there's something wrong with it.'

'Says that to everybody.'

'Aye, well. I want you around just in case there's any shenanigans.'

'Shenanigans there won't be.'

By this time we were at Edward's door. Pamela knocked and opened it. Edward was sitting at his table, totting up rows of figures.

'Edward, you wanted me to have a look at you?'

'Oh aye,' said Edward and put away his sums. He stood up from the table.

'I've brought Dennis with me.'

'Aye, okay.' Edward didn't bother. The more the merrier.

I stood with my back to the door, blocking the little window so nobody could look in. Pamela moved to the far wall so that Edward would be obliged to turn his back on the door, thereby ensuring a little more privacy. Then she said, 'All right,' and nodded at the region of his groin. Edward unbelted his trousers and pulled them and his pants down to his knees.

Pamela was too good a nurse to say or do anything unprofessional. Edward probably didn't notice, but I did. I've rarely seen eyes go quite that large that quickly. I chewed my lip. Pamela's expression was one of complete professionalism.

'What do you think is wrong with it?' she said.

'It's red, there. Look.'

'Yes,' said Pamela shortly, motioning to him to pull his kecks back up and moving away, 'and we know what's doing that, don't we?'

Edward looked puzzled. But he got dressed. We left, me closing the door behind us.

Pamela, a married lady, waited till we were well down the corridor and on our own.

'Nothing wrong with that,' she said.

'My thoughts entirely,' I agreed.

'It's an ill-divided world,' she said with a smile.

'So they say,' I said.

Increased libido is a characteristic of the manic state. Maybe Edward's perpetual showing off of his wares was a sublimation of it. The next thing he did was not sublimated. It was about as direct and unsublimated as you can get.

A young woman was admitted a week or two after Edward, off her rocker with a drug-induced psychosis. We were not unused to her type of presentation, singing and dancing around, but it was not common. After four or five days she was starting to show real signs of recovery and was close to being discharged.

Morning time. The first batch of the shift had been in for the night duty report from Geraldine. Next up were Luke, John, Clyde and me. The others went about the morning routine on the ward. One fetched in the trolley; one opened up the kitchen; Pamela went to the Treatment Room to arrange morning meds, and Gordon went round the doors.

He came fairly quickly, and fairly red-faced, back to the office.

'You'll need tae have a word wi' Edward an' that lassie.'

'What lassie?' said Geraldine.

'The new lassie.'

'What's been going on?' said Geraldine, her voice taking on a barbed edge.

'I went into the lassie's room tae tell her it was breakfast, and they were at it.'

'At it? Having sex?'

'Well naw. Well, aye, but no actual . . . you ken . . .'

'What were they doing, Gordon?'

'Ah don't like tae say. She was lying back oan the bed an' . . . well, ye ken.'

'Right!'

Geraldine stood up and stalked off. I didn't fancy being either Edward or the new lassie. Gordon smirked at us blokes.

'Edward was goin' at her like a dug eatin' stovies,' he said.

'Too much information, man,' said Clyde.

'As well Geraldine didn't hear that, Gordo,' said Luke. 'Else your feet wouldn't have touched.'

'I only meant . . .'

'Time and place, Gordy, time and place,' said Luke as we went out into the ward.

'Forsooth,' I said in my best Maggie Smith voice, 'one should have a sense of these things.'

I don't know exactly what Geraldine said to Edward but he was fairly quiet for . . . oh, almost an hour, as a result. He did his race walk around the courtyard and came back in silence, heading through to his room and speaking to no one. The young woman stayed in her room for most of the day. Alone. As I say, I don't know what was said, but I envied neither of the guilty parties. Geraldine was a formidable woman. Nobody crossed her lightly or fucked around on her watch.

I was out in the courtyard later in the day, enjoying some sunlight and a wheeze with a few of the patients when Edward came out.

'Hi, Dennis,' he said. 'Hi. Got a light? Gimme a light, please. Thanks. Great, you're a pal.'

'How you feelin' now, man?' I said.

'In the pink, Dennis, in the pink.'

'Got over that bollocking Geraldine gave you?'

'Wow! What a woman, what a woman. She was angry all right. Tore strips off me, tore strips. I just told her that it was nothin' to get uptight about, you know what I mean, nothing to get agitated about. I said we were just gettin' it on.'

'Just a lover and his lass, with a hey and a ho.'

'I don't know what that means, Dennis, but it's no against the law, know what I mean? No against the law. That's what I told her.'

'Oh aye, I bet Geraldine was amused at that.'

'No too, tae be honest, Dennis. No too. She told me it was . . . what was the word? Inappropriate, that was it. Inappropriate. And that I was takin' advantage ae the lassie's condition. Well, I didnae take advantage ae anybody. She was the one that pulled me ontae the bed.'

'We'll leave it there, I think.'

'Geraldine's an angry woman. An angry woman.'

'I take it she made it clear there was to be no repeats.'

'No! No repeats. Else she said I'd end up on close obs. I dinnae want that, Dennis. Dinnae want that.'

'No, of course you don't. You'll need to stop showin' off your mighty Wurlitzer to folk,' I suggested.

'No showin' it aff, Dennis. Ahm no a show-aff. Ahm just proud ae a mah manhood.'

'That's not your manhood, Eddie baby,' I said. 'That's just your cock. Never confuse the two.'

He looked at me, puzzled. I left him to think about it.

Theo had taken to wearing a watch. I'd never seen him with one before, but all of a sudden he appeared one day with one on. It was a metal bracelet watch, only Theo didn't wear it on his wrist. He wore it halfway up his arm, around his bicep. We are so used to seeing someone turn their wrist up to their gaze when asked the time. It's quite a difference to see someone shove his wrist behind his head and consult his bicep. That's what Theo did.

'Where'd you get the watch, Theo?' said John.

'In my things. Forgot I had it, but I found it going through my things. Been there for ages.'

'Why'd you wear it up there?'

'It was my father's.'

John looked nonplussed for a moment.

'Forgive me, Theo,' he said, 'but I believe that is what's called a non sequitur.'

'No, man,' said Theo. 'It's an Ingersoll.'

He came into the Smoke Room one day as I sat looking out the window and pondering deeply upon the vicissitudes of fate. Bill was there too.

'Hey, man,' Theo said to me. 'Have you seen Edward's cock?'

'Why? Has he lost it?' said Bill.

'Yeah, very good, man,' Theo said. Then he addressed me again: 'No, I mean seriously, have you seen it?'

'I should think most of the hospital have seen it by now.'

'It's ridiculous. His cock soft is bigger than my cock hard.'

'As a very shrewd woman once said, Theo, it's an ill-divided world.'

'Ain't that the truth.'

And away he went.

But I'm not quite done with Edward and his sexuality. A day or two after he was discovered in flagrante, he nabbed me in the Laundry Room. I'd been showing some ditsy young dame where to put the powder and the water and her washing in the machine, when Edward wandered in.

He waited till the girl had gone and then collared me as I made to leave.

'Can I ask your advice, Dennis? Need to ask you something. That okay? That all right?'

'I'm not looking at your penis, Edward.'

'Ha ha. That's very funny. No, no, not that. Not that. I need your advice.'

'Okay, I'll buy it,' I said. 'What is it?'

'Do you think I should go gay?'

'Go? Gay?'

'Aye. Do you think I should, eh? Go gay. Go gay.'

'I'm not sure that gay is somewhere you can go, Eddie baby. I think you're either there or you're not.'

'Ah but, Geraldine, you know Geraldine?'

'Yes.'

'She said I hadn't to do anything wi' the lassie again. Not to do anything sexual with her. An' she was right up for it. She was keener than me. Anyway, anyway, don't give me a row. I'm not sayin' anythin' against her. A man's got his urges, Dennis. Know what I mean? That's all I'm sayin'. And if I can't have a woman's love, well . . . Should I go gay?'

'Why?'

'It's either that or die of chronic masturbation.'

'And what do you think would happen if you went gay? That one of the blokes in here would welcome you into his cold little bed? I think Geraldine would have something to say about that an' all.'

'Hah! You're right. She would, she would. She'd go through me like a dose of salts.'

'There you are then. Not worth it.'

'What should I do?'

'If I were you, Eduardo, I should wait patiently until you're discharged from here and then I should play the tomcat with all those fine dames in the big city.'

'Yeah! That's it! I will, I will. Thanks, Dennis, you're a pal.'

'Okay, pal. Fancy a coffee? You do? Let's do it.'

Why should we assume that young healthy people shouldn't be interested in sex, shouldn't have the urge or shouldn't try and do something about it, just because they're temporarily incarcerated in a locked ward? I don't think libido works like that. Certainly Edward's didn't.

27

Home is the sailor, home from the sea,
And the hunter home from the hill.
Robert Louis Stevenson, 'Requiem'

One of the great moments in a patient's stay on the Locked Ward was when he or she was allowed out of the hospital grounds. The pattern was generally a half-hour's escorted walk in the grounds for a time, to establish that the patient was all right with the whiff of fresh air and not liable to bolt like a rabbit. If that went without any hitches, the patient might be allowed unescorted time out of the ward, only half an hour again at first, time enough to get to the garage for ciggies and back. Gradually, all being well, the time would increase until, just before discharge, they might be allowed a weekend back home with parents or spouse, to see how that went. There were many variations on this, of course, but that was the basic pattern.

From time to time a patient would request a trip to the town shops to buy clothes or a CD player, something that wasn't readily available either in the hospital shop or the filling station. This was granted at Charlie's discretion. If the ward was relatively quiet, and the staffing complement relatively sound, he would sometimes ask one of us to take a patient to the town centre.

'Dennis, Edward's needing some togs. Fancy getting a hospital car and driving him to the centre?'

Oh yessiree, Chuck, I'm your man. I don't know about the rest of the staff but I looked on time out of the ward like a schoolboy looks on time out of class. A jape. A jamboree. Playing hookey. Plugging it, as they said when I was at school. That was a long time ago, certainly, about the time of the Second Jacobite Rebellion, and the term may have fallen out of use. But the feeling was familiar from days of old. I think I enjoyed those times out more than some of the patients did.

Summertime had come. If the living had not yet reached the easy stage, the fish not yet fully fit for jumping, nor the cotton in a state of sufficient altitude, it could not be denied that the clocks were well forward and had been for months. The air was pleasanter, allegro non molto in G minor. Here and there, in glade and copse, bees that had forgotten the words were starting to hum. Birds were clearing their throats in preparation for singing to consumptive poets. Charlie spoke to me over breakfast one morning and uttered the very sentences that you'll find some 200 words back in the text. I was nothing loth. Whatever that means.

To get a hospital car meant having to seek a favour from the porters. They had a wee lodge near the entrance to the hospital and a supplicant had to approach this on his knees from a distance of a hundred yards down the corridor, all the while beating his breast and intoning in plain chant, '*Non sum dignus, non sum dignus.*' On arriving at the entrance to the Porters' Lodge – the porters' portal – the supplicant was required to prostrate himself upon the threshold and cry, 'May the all-powerful porters grant a humbler life form a hearing, in their almighty goodness and generosity!' Only then could the supplicant stand up and await the porters' mighty doom.

'What the fuck do *you* want?' was the usual retort when one woke a busy porter.

'I was hoping you might be able to find me a hospital car.'

'A car! He wants a car!' he would guffaw. As if the request was the single most ludicrous thing he had heard all day, a request as outlandish as asking for a barouche, or a square-rigged merchant ship of the 1850s.

'Have you got one that I could borrow for an hour?'

'Ah. Well. I'll need to see. For an oor, you say? Could maybe manage that. If it's back in an oor.'

'Aye, well, just to take a patient to the centre, buy some shit and come back.'

'Oh aye. You're fae 25, int ye?'

'I am, yes.'

'I'll see if there's wan free. Ye see, aw they cars is booked oot. Regular. Booked oot, ye see.'

He approached a shelf where the folders pertaining to the pool of hospital cars were kept. I expected to see one battered blue folder lying forgotten, on its side, if I were lucky. There were at least five. So not all of them were booked oot. Rats were smelt. He lifted a folder and handed it to me gracelessly.

'Effin' cee,' he said. I thought this was a bit thick. All I wanted was a car.

'How d'you mean?' I said, prepared to be vexed if the occasion warranted it.

'FNC,' he enunciated, as if he were addressing a simpleton. 'That's the car reg. It's a blue Modus. You'll find it in the car park. Mind – an oor.'

I thanked him profusely and exited from the lodge backwards, bowing and genuflecting as I went. I found it in the car park, a slightly crusty vehicle with a stale guff in it, as of last Saturday's takeaway and fumble. It was, nonetheless, a car. I put on my cap and my string-backed gloves, then tooled it round the hospital to Ward 25 and tooted on the horn. Edward appeared after a minute's delay, beaming like a lighthouse. He packed himself into the passenger seat.

'Right, Dennis. This is great. Let's go, let's go, get the pedal tae the metal. You know the drill. If we hit anybody just keep drivin'. If anybody hits us, we'll get out an' lamp them. Okay, let's GO!'

I looked at him. He smiled sweetly.

'I'll shut up, will I?' he said.

'Well, if you would . . .'

He shut up and I pulled away.

'This is great, Dennis, great. Wonderful. Marvellous. In the pink, in the pink.'

'Shut the fuck up, Eddie, or we're going nowhere.'

'Mum's the word. You can rely on me. I just need a couple of shirts and a pair of jeans. Just shirts and jeans.'

He never halted his rattle all the way to the town centre, all the way from the parked car to the shops, or all the way around the shops. But I forgave him. He was as excited as a schoolboy. I wasn't far short of it. We went into a supermarket with a big clothes section.

'Lots a clothes in here, Dennis. Tons a clothes.'

'Yes. Quite reasonable too. And not shite for the price.'

'Aye, aye. You're right, you're right.'

He stopped at the women's section and started to hold out tops from a circular rack.

'Lovely colours, Dennis, eh? Beautiful. Lovely colours. Fair envy the girls sometimes, some of the clothes they get to wear, eh?'

'You're no goin' tranny on me, are you?'

'Nnnnnaaaw!' he scoffed. 'Just like the colours. Where's the shirts?'

'You usually find them in the men's section.'

'Ha! You're on the ball the day, Den, on the ball the day.'

We found the men's section and he flitted around the racks of shirts like a moth. Meanwhile I leaned against a wall and tried to look detached and Byronic, yet at the same time warm and witty if only you could get to the real me underneath. Eventually he came over carrying two garments so garish I wouldn't have hung them as curtains in a North African knocking shop.

'Do you think these'll suit me, Dennis?'

'You goin' to a fancy dress party?'

'D'you not like them?'

'You'd be better with some of the blouses you were looking at earlier.'

'Och, they're no that bad, no that bad. This one – checked shirt. *You* wear checked shirts.'

'Sometimes, yeah. But the check is wee. Quiet. That looks like you lifted it off a table in a Greek restaurant.'

'Does it?' His look of disappointment shamed me.

'C'mere,' I said and led him back to the racks. 'There – that one. How about that one? Checked but no screaming the place down.'

'Aye! Aye! I like that. How much is that?'

I checked the tag.

'You can get two shirts off that rack for a tenner.'

'That's good, isn't it, that's good. Let me see. What about that one?'

'Yeah. If you like that. That's cool.'

He had picked a plain dark-blue cotton.

'I like that. Like that. That'd go well wae my new jeans.'

'So it would. Now you're talkin' wi' gas. What size are you?'

'Medium.'

'Okay. Look at the wee coloured squares on the hangers. Tells you the size. You're looking for a capital M. That means medium. That one you've got there would fit Hoss Cartwright. Look – XL. What the hell would you want an XL shirt for? It'd look like a smock on you.'

'Who's Hoss Cartwright?'

'Pal o' mine. Right. Got two mediums?'

'Should that no be two "media"?'

'Good, Edward. Yeah, very good. Okay, let's get the jeans.'

He took the two shirts and dropped them in a basket. Then he picked a pair of blue jeans. We stood in the checkout queue. The girl beeping a woman's shopping over the scanner was young but as stone-faced as Ozymandias. This did not deter Edward from beaming and winking at her any time she looked up from her work. She was not impressed by his attentions.

'Heh, sir,' I whispered. 'Control yourself.'

'Just bein' nice, Dennis. Just bein' nice.'

Then it was our turn. She took the two shirts and flapped them, ran them over the scanner, then folded them up.

'You've done that before, hen,' said Edward. 'I can tell by the way you're doin' it. Skilful, like. You've got the tech-knack.'

Now, much to my chagrin, she smiled. His cheesy old patter had made her smile.

'And the jeans tae, hen. That's the game. Now, don't you be imaginin' how mah backside would look in theym. Your boyfriend'll get jealous.'

Now she giggled.

'Nae boyfriend,' she said and blushed slightly. This was sick-making.

'Nae boyfriend? I'm no believin' that. Good-lookin' girl like you. Good-lookin' girl like you. Bet you're batterin' them away wi' a golf club.'

'Come on, Ed,' I interrupted, looking at my watch. 'We'll need to get back to the hospital. Get that car back.'

'Oh,' the girl said, stopping and looking at us. 'Are youse fae the hospital?'

Edward didn't miss a beat.

'Aye. He likes to get oot for a wee while every day, just to get oot the ward. So I drive him around wae me when I'm daein' mah shoppin' and things like that. But he's daein' well. He'll be gettin' hame soon.'

I didn't say anything to this. I couldn't. I was laughing too much. Finessed. Trumped. Outmanoeuvred, outdone and outplayed. A quick piece of thinking.

He insisted on buying a magazine at the news counter before we left. I dallied in the foyer while he did, and then we went back to the hospital. I dropped him at the ward and returned the car to the porters, with accompanying grovels and tributes, before I made my own way back to 25.

Edward was in the main corridor, pirouetting like a mannequin in his new blue shirt and jeans for the adoration of the assembled throng.

'Very smart, Edward,' said Geraldine as she passed.

'Yeah, nice duds, man,' said Theo.

'You look very nice,' added a female patient.

'Come and see what else I got, Dennis,' said Edward when I arrived at the catwalk.

'I was there, Ed. I saw it all.'

'No, come and see this.'

He took me along to his room and there, on the wall above his bed he had Blu-tacked one of those naff little jokey cards. He showed it off with a sweeping gesture of his arm like a guide in an art gallery: YOU DON'T HAVE TO BE MAD TO WORK HERE BUT IT HELPS. I smiled.

'Making a point, Edward?'

'Just a jokey one, Dennis, just a jokey one.'

'You know how to tell the difference between the patients and the staff in here?' I said.

'No. Tell me, Dennis. Is it a joke, is it a joke?'

'The patients get better and go away,' I said. 'The staff get worse and stay on.'

He liked that.

Our little excursion had gone so well that I drove him through to the city the following week. He had been saying to Charlie that he would like to get home and check his mail, see if there was a cheque from the benefits office. I got that gig too.

I tooled old FNC out the back roads to the city, taking the scenic route to spin the trip out. We listened to the in-car entertainment system and smoked our lungs sooty. The miles went by quietly as a blameless life. Needless to say, Edward burbled and chattered for the entire journey, radio or not, but I didn't bother. Shits were not given that day. The weather was fair; time was not pressing. A wireless set near to bring us some cheer, as somebody who wasn't Shakespeare once said.

Edward had a flat in a suburb in the south of the city, the middle apartment of three in one side of a tenement block. It was a late 1950s, early '60s development, so not too eye-catching in the architecture department, but it seemed a quiet and respectable area. Trim gardens, neat lawns, smartly painted front doors, UPVC replacement windows. No litter. One old guy in a hat walking his dog.

'Seems like a nice area, Eddie baby,' I said as we pulled up outside his block. 'Quiet.'

'Too quiet. Too quiet for me, Dennis. It's like a cemetery, a cemetery.'

We piled out of the bucket and entered the tenement. I could have sworn several lace curtains fell back into place as we did. Up the stairs to the second landing. Edward's door on the left-hand side. He unlocked it and had to shove it open, against the drift of post behind it.

'Someb'dy loves you,' I said.

'Hope the benefits people do,' he said.

I helped him to lift the mail. Armfuls of it each. We carried it through to the living room and he cascaded his lot onto the settee. I followed suit. Edward sat down and began to go through it.

'Have a look round, Dennis. Help yourself. Feel free. *Mi casa su casa* and all that. There might be some coffee in the cupboard. There's maybe milk in the fridge.'

'If there is, it'll be green cheese by now.'

'Ha ha ha. You're right, you're right.'

I wandered through to the kitchen. It was all very neat and tidy, much more so than I'd expected. The worktops were spotless. On one there was a circular bread board on its rim against the wall and a mug tree. Taps and kettle gleaming. Fridge whitely humming. I opened it. Nothing. I found a jar of coffee in a cupboard and made a drink for Edward. I took it back through to him. He was ripping envelopes open with a finger, scanning the contents and discarding the letters at his feet.

'Here. Black coffee.'

'Ta, Dennis, ta very much. Not having one yourself?'

'I'm okay. These the letters you've read?' I asked, nodding at the pile on the floor.

'Aye, ha ha. Read letter day.'

'You keep yourself awfully spick and span here for a young buck with no baggage. I thought you were strictly rock 'n' roll. A night rider on the road to perdition. A wild babbling hard-on on legs.'

'My mum comes in once a week and tidies up.'

That figured. It looked like it had been given a loving mother's touch. I wandered through the rest of the flat. Bathroom spotless. Bedroom similar with a double bed all neatly made up, and the carpet hoovered to within an inch of its shagpile. It could have been the home of some respectable widowed lady of the parish. Gordon's Imogen, in fact. Then I opened the other bedroom door. It was completely bare – walls, floorboards, uncurtained windows – and empty save for a drum kit right in the middle of the floor. A double-bass-drum kit, with two standing toms, in black sparkle, with a forest of crash and ride cymbals surrounding it. I'd forgotten that Edward used to be a drummer in a band. I strolled through to the living room again.

'Some kit you got there, man,' I said.

'Yeah, it's cool, isn't it, Dennis? Cool. Look!' He waved a letter in the air. 'That's what I was looking for. My cheque's through.'

'Good. You play the drums a lot?'

'Practise every night. At least an hour. Sometimes more. Sometimes lots more. Hours at times.'

'I bet the neighbours are highly amused at that.'

'No, they don't like it, Dennis. Don't like it. Always complaining. Never away from the door.'

'I'm surprised at that. Anyway, got what you wanted? We'll tidy up this paper trail and head back to the Happy House.'

'Naw, naw. Leave it, leave it, Dennis. Mum'll do it. Mum'll do it. She's better at it than me. I'll phone her tonight. She'll get it in a bin liner.'

I shrugged.

Edward said, 'I'll give you a blast on the kit before we go.'

He did. He sat on the stool behind the battery of percussion instruments and played. Played very well, as a matter of fact, thundering rolls and sharp staccato rhythms. But the noise was appalling. In that little cell of a room, stripped of everything that might have been calculated to deaden sound, it felt like the entire house was coming down about our ears. I waved at him after two minutes. He rumbled to a stop.

'Right, enough! You're damned good, but the noise is deafening. No wonder the neighbours kick up fuck.'

'Always, Dennis. Never happy. One time in the summer I stripped the kit down and carried it out onto the back green. Set it up out there. Nice sound, with all the walls around me. Like in the courtyard at the ward, just like the courtyard.'

'Yeah. I bet everybody was entertained at that.'

'They sent for the police. Can you believe it? Sent for the police.'

'Oh, I can believe it all right.'

We locked up, leaving the mail for Edward's mother, and tripped back down the stairs and out into the car. Lace curtains *definitely* fell this time. As we pulled away, I thought I saw old folk emerge from their doors and commence dancing in the street and setting off fireworks.

I took Theo home about this time too, and he elicited much the same reaction from his neighbours as Edward had done in the city. Only Theo lived in the town. Five minutes' drive from the ward. We parked in front of the flats where he kept his abode.

'That old dude in the garden, man,' said Theo, 'he's uncool and heavy. He's got no time for heads or the Dharma Bums. Totally uncool and fucked up.'

We got out of the car and the old man looked up from his hoeing. He got his eyes on us and I've never seen a human being get so sad so quickly. Theo was obviously the last one he wanted to see. He stood and watched as we approached the flats, then with a disgusted shake of his head turned away.

'See what I mean, man? You dig?'

I dug. The elderly gent was obviously unaware that Theo was a hipster and a head, not to mention golden billion-year-old carbon. Or, if he was aware of it, it didn't impress him much. Into the tenement we went. Theo was on the top floor. His pad was a revelation.

Unlike Edward's, Theo's place had never seen the bristle of a brush since the days of Old King Tut. Dust lay in dunes along the lino and thickly drifted on every conceivable surface: sills, shelves, tabletops, chairs. His living-room wall was covered in posters of rock events, prints of album covers, the kind of soft porn art beloved of single stags and one huge psychedelically coloured mandala. There were piles of papers and magazines, and scattered cups and plates, none of which was remotely clean. Ashtrays were everywhere. Some of the flicked ash had actually landed somewhere near some of them. And shelves and shelves of New Age memorabilia: runes, wooden joss burners, a tarot pack, candles, at least a dozen brass skulls of varying sizes, goblets and a large metal pentagram on a chain. I was walking into the opening chords of an Incredible String Band LP.

Now Theo materialised by my side. He opened his fist and there, in the palm of his hand, lay a small piece of stone. It was a greyish-creamy colour, like a chip of sandstone. I looked at it carefully, as I was obviously expected to do, and then looked up at him.

'Do you know what this is?' he said.

'I don't know, Theo. Another piece of kryptonite?'

He laughed. 'Better.'

'Better than kryptonite? I don't know . . .'

'It's a piece of Stonehenge. I chipped it off one of the triliths one summer evening long ago. It has magical qualities.'

'Heavy thing to do, man,' I said. 'What was it you told Edward about not taking anything off Ayers Rock? Brings a curse.'

'That's Uluru, man. Different vibe entirely. It's sacred to the Aborigines. Stonehenge is worshipped by Druids. Groovy people. Stardust. Not at all the same thing.'

I was suitably enlightened.

'Yeah. I chipped that off Stonehenge, and then this chick and I climbed Glastonbury Tor and balled at midnight. It was exceptionally mellow, man.'

But the most memorable part of Theo's flat – I didn't risk the bedroom – was the kitchen. The door was closed but it seemed to me that there was a distinct hum coming from behind it. Let me rephrase that. There were *two* distinct hums coming from behind it, one of the traditional aural variety, the other concentrating more on the olfactory system.

'What's in there, Theo?'

'The kitchen, man.'

I opened the door. The air was a soup of flies. I closed it again extremely quickly, but still had time to notice the alp of litter and garbage that sloped down the far wall.

'You've got the fourth plague of Egypt going on in your fucking kitchen, man,' I said.

'What?'

'Your collection of flies is doing well,' I said.

'What, man? Surely they're dead by now.'

'The original ones might be, but their grandchildren are doing well. What's that heap of shit and crud you've got in the corner? You can't just toss your refuse away in the house.'

'Hey, chill, man. It's only paper – you know, boxes and packages, man. Can't do any harm.'

'Yes, it can. It'll have fragments of stuff in it. Encourage vermin. Those flies will be laying eggs all over the shit. There'll be maggots . . . ach!'

'Drop down a gear, man. Once in a while I get a big bag and bag it all up, give the place a spring clean, you know?'

'Once in a while? About as often as Halley's comet, probably. We need to do something about this. Unless you want Environmental Health evicting you for being a polluted get.'

Theo refused to discuss the matter any more. He too found the cheque he was looking for. Meanwhile I picked a reasonably uninfected spot in the carpet and stayed there. The rest of this tip I did not wish to see.

The following day Luke and I returned with Theo and several stout black refuse bags. Once we'd opened the window and unleashed the cloud of flies on the locality, it was the work of half an hour to bag up the shit and toss it in a skip. Which was just as well. Plan B had been to paint a huge red cross on the front door and toss a canister of Zyklon B into the fucking place.

How different, as they say, from the home life of our own dear Queen.

28

Why, this is lunatics! This is mad as a mad dog!
William Shakespeare, *The Merry Wives of Windsor*

I had had my summer vacation. Two weeks away from the Locked Ward, out in the sane world where recession sent the value of sterling plummeting to roughly the equivalent of a string of beads; where the planet was heating up like a gas ring; where babies were abused in nurseries and children killed by aerial bombardment in the Middle East; where suicide bombers and stray missiles killed the innocent at home, at work and play – war, torture, poverty and death. Just a normal two weeks in the outside world.

When I parked the old jalopy outside the ward on my first morning back, Luke and John were holding the outside door open for two male nurses from 24, Ronnie and Andy. When we got into the ward itself, besides those four and myself, there were Charlie, Gordon and Clyde, as well as our usual complement of female colleagues. Eight males. Four females. Either the top brass were planning to train staff in the Dashing White Sergeant as a new form of therapy, or there was a 'handful' on the ward. (A 'handful' was the understated term favoured by Charlie to denote a particularly violent individual, or one who required extra personnel while being restrained.)

John filled us in while we removed our jackets in the Locker Room.

'The other shift phoned me yesterday afternoon. See if I could come in and give them handers. New admission goin' doolally, needed a bit of extra muscle. Got here, and there was three guys in from 24 – Andy, Ronnie and Tosh.'

'Ho, we got a handful?' I said.

'A belter, Denny. A belter. Polis brought the guy in – local guy – cuffed up and angry. Took the bracelets aff 'im an' he went for it. Big style. Broke Jake's nose.'

'Fucksake!'

'Yeah,' said Ronnie. 'Took four of us to hold him. But not before he put the head on Jake and bust his snitch.'

'Know 'im?' I asked.

'Na,' said John. 'New one to me. Terry somethin'.'

We took the report from Charlie that morning with six men in the office. The other two stayed up at the station because the new man, having been restrained and jagged at three in the morning, was sleeping that one off. It was felt that we could risk six being away from the vicinity of his room. Charlie told us that this was a first presentation, and that he was in his twenties, lived with his parents and had become increasingly withdrawn and self-isolating at home. He had a good job in one of the factories on the nearby industrial estate but was in danger of losing it because of his increasingly frequent absences.

'If Dr Marjorie slaps a longer section on him, that's him covered. Doctor's line,' said Gordon. 'You know – a sick note.'

'Well, yeah, thanks for that,' said Charlie. 'Anyway. Guy has no girlfriend. Was going with a lassie for two years and she dumped him. May be the source of the problems.

Recently taken to verbal aggression with his old folks. Which worried them, of course. Taking things to a new level. Tried to persuade him to see the GP; was having none of it. Night before last got pissed out his brain and started to rant and rave at his father. Father's about fifty-eight or fifty-nine. Father remonstrated; Terry lashed out with some kind of poker thing and just missed taking the old man's block off. Went berserk, smashing the place up. The folks called the police. He got huckled and brought here. Thomas was duty doc and sectioned him. And he is a handful. Instantly and constantly enraged. Been restrained six times and jagged. Sleeps it off, just keeps coming again.'

This I did not find comforting. Oh, restraints were no big deal to me by that time. I had been restraining like a bastard with the guys, whichever guys were around, for some time. Got a little blasé about it, to be frank. Somewhat disentranced by the whole process. But it was some time since we'd had a handful. To be honest, I couldn't remember the last one. I thought it rather amusing that Thomas had sectioned him, though. Thomas was the SHO at that time, and a more constantly enraged man it would be hard to imagine. Luke said Thomas had given him a lift one winter morning after his own car broke down. Snow was whirling. The man in the car in front was driving carefully, since his back end kept fishtailing in the snow. Thomas tailgated him, sitting on his arse all the way to the hospital turn-off, growing increasingly red in the face and bellowing at intervals, 'This is the kind of arsehole that causes ACCIDENTS!'

It was just after lunchtime when Terry Somethin' surfaced. He had missed breakfast as well as lunch. The twelve of us had found it difficult to think of enough things to do in the meanwhile. Patients were offered walks, games of cards, shots on the computer, the chance to play the guitar or the organ in the GP Room and assorted other pastimes, several times an hour by several people. They were all activitied out. No fewer than four males stayed around the station area at any time. Every once in a while someone would walk over and look through the window in his door.

'Still out.'

'Drivin' the pigs home.'

'Sleepin' like a baby.'

Then it was my turn. I came up the ward from having a fag in the Smoke Room and cast an insouciant eye through the Judas window. The bed was empty.

'He's not in his farter,' I said.

Everyone scrambled. There were six men on their feet in an instant. I looked through the window slightly from the side so that I could see into the lavatory. He was standing at the pan.

'He's takin' a slash,' I said.

'Keep the bulletins comin',' said Luke.

'Now he's washin' his hands.'

'I was jokin', Dennis. Will you come to fuck away from there?'

This was not Lukelike. There was an edge to his voice. Everybody was tensed, on the balls of their feet. I needed no second bidding, however. I came to fuck away from there. I'm not sorry I did.

The door opened and he came out. Terry Somethin' did not *look* like a handful. In fact, he looked like he couldn't fight sleep. He had a round little face with a gooseberry growth of beard and sported a noticeable pot.

But he was a handful, all right. He was game. Game as five-a-sides. Game as Monopoly. Game as three brace of pheasant that have been hanging in the back lobby for a fortnight.

John faced him. 'You hungry, Terry? You've missed breakfast and lunch. We can do you something to eat.'

Terry's face darkened as recognition dawned. His lips slid back and he bared his teeth.

'You, ya bastard!' he hissed. 'You done me yesterday, didn't ye?'

And he leaped at John, who was taken by surprise. Terry was already astride him when he hit the floor, flurrying punches at his face. Luke, Clyde and Ronnie dived as a pack on Terry. I set off my alarm as two of the other patients came running to see what was happening.

'Okay, guys,' I shouted. 'Vacate the area just now. Restraint going on. Go away till it's done.'

'Vacate fuck all,' screamed one guy, a malcontent from the city named Bryce. 'Leave him alone, you Nazi bastards!' And he swung a vicious kick that connected with Clyde about halfway up his back.

As Clyde yelled in pain and I grabbed Bryce by one arm, Andy taking the other, Gordon came running up the ward with Charlie and Pamela.

'Draw it up, Pam,' said Charlie and helped us to deck Bryce, putting him into the position.

Pamela sprinted off to the Treatment Room. The second patient, a man in his forties, screamed at the top of his voice, 'They're killin' them! Killin' them!' and swung a roundhouse punch at me. A skilled fighter would have seen it coming from a week last Tuesday. I'm not a skilled fighter. It struck me flush on the boko, and I squealed like a big lassie. Blood flowed. I rolled off Bryce, and Gordon at once jumped into my place.

The floor by now was pandemonium, with the drub of running feet and the calls of alarmed patients. Terry was still shrieking benedictions upon his restrainers at the top of his voice. Bryce was shouting about Nazis and bully boys. Patients were milling about, asking what was going on, saying we couldn't do that; it was against the law, goading each other on to intervene. More male staff arrived – somebody had obviously put out a Treble Three – and the patient who had hit me was huckled away. Charlie was yelling at Geraldine to get a jag drawn up for Bryce as well as Terry. And I was staggering about like a sheep with the scrapie. My nose was pishing blood and my eyes were pishing water.

Gentle, kindly, female hands led me to a seat.

'Sit down, Dennis, let me see . . .' It was a staff nurse from 24, a lovely big woman called Jessie. She had a quick squint at my neb and reassured me. 'Hold your head back and pinch on the bridge of your nose . . . higher up . . . at the nasal root . . .'

I wasn't au fait with the geography of the human beak but common sense told me where to pinch it.

'That's it. Hold it there and you'll be right as rain in no time.'

'What happened, man?' asked Theo, stepping in as Jessie moved out.

'Got pudged od the dose.'

'Heavy, man. What the fuck is all this scene about? It's like the fight in *Seven Brides for Seven Brothers*.'

'Theo, you aren't progressing things here at the moment,' called Charlie from the floor. 'Folks, can you move the patients out down the corridor and lock off this bedded area?'

'You got it, Chas,' called a male voice, and started to head 'em up and move 'em out.

In short order the area was closed off. Then began the jabbing. Pamela gave Terry his injection, Terry all the while calling down the blessings of heaven upon her for being such an angel. Geraldine spiked Bryce and asked Charlie if my assailant was to be done too.

'Offer him it orally,' decided Charlie. 'If he refuses, we'll jag him too.'

After some time Terry had subsided enough to permit the guys to raise him ever so gently to his feet and escort him back into his room.

'Stay in here, Terry,' advised Charlie, 'and we'll bring you something to eat.'

'Fuck you! You can't keep me here against my will.'

'We can and we are going to,' Charlie contradicted him. 'You're sectioned under the Mental Health Act. You have to stay here until our consultant thinks you're ready to go home again.'

'You're gonna regret that,' threatened Terry. 'Your orderlies are gonna get their fuckin' heads kicked in every time they come near me.'

'And you'll be restrained and given an intramuscular injection every time you assault a member of my staff. They're here to help you, not to be assaulted. By you or by anybody else.'

'How can these bastards help *me*? They don't know me.'

'We know enough about you and about the illness you're suffering from at the moment to know how to nurse you.

Just give us the chance to do it and we'll get you out of here and back home as quickly as we can.'

Bryce was returned to his room and advised to take a time-out to reflect upon his earlier behaviour. The guy who had given me a red nose had taken oral meds and, reflecting that discretion is the better part of valour, had gone to his room and lain down. John had a black eye and a swollen lip. Clyde had a lump on his back and the first signs of some serious bruising, but nothing was broken. My nose had stopped bleeding, and I looked like W. C. Fields after a night on the Ol' Red Eye.

Once Terry had eaten and was asleep again, most of us gathered in the office. John and Ronnie, who was a big hulker of a guy, stayed up the business end of the ward in case the Porteous Riots kicked off again.

'Well done, people,' said Charlie. 'That was a difficult situation, and you handled it well. Clyde's okay; John's got a sore face but it won't affect his pulling power any; and the old boy here . . .' he smiled at me '. . . will soon look like his usual frisky self again. You did well. Terry's zonked again. Bryce is taking some time to chill.'

'That's a bad bastard,' said Luke. 'I know Terry's not well – we all know that – but Bryce is just an opportunist. He just took the chance to kick a member of staff when they were busy.'

'He's ill as well, Luke, or he wouldn't be here. It's hard to remember that sometimes when things like this happen. But that's what we have to remember. That's why we're in this ward. To help guys like these. Not always easy, I grant you. But we have to try at all times.'

'I see what Luke beads, though, Charlie,' I said. 'Because folk are id here, it doesd't bead they're dot the sabe as they are outside. Like there's good guys add bad bastards out there; there's good guys add bad bastards id here too.'

Charlie smiled.

'Melvyn Bragg meets Timothy Leary,' he said. 'I know what you mean, Dennis. But it's still true. Unconditional care. That's what we're here for.'

I don't know that anybody ever expressed it better. Charlie had his critics among some staff – who doesn't? Some thought he was a dinosaur because he'd been in his post for years and years. Some felt that on his watch the ethos of the Locked Ward had become macho, drenched in testosterone. There was a perception among some staff external to the ward that we were too ready with the physical restraint and the needle. This was wholly wrong and a grave calumny on Charlie. He was at all times a skilled and caring nurse, with a wealth of experience that he brought to bear on every situation. And he ran a good ward. Patients liked him; staff liked him. He had each individual patient's welfare in the forefront of his mind at all times. You can't praise a nurse much more than that.

In time Terry calmed down. There even came a time when he could walk out of his room without flying at the first nurse he saw. He called me Jim. I don't know why. But he was not the only one to call me a different name. Bill, of the imaginative dress sense and the rap poetry, rarely called anyone by their given name. For whatever reason, I was Paddy. I met him on a street in the town one time when he was out of the ward and he beamed at me and said, 'Hi, Paddy. Still banged up in that hoaspital?'

Terry got calmer, like I say, but never quite lost the itch to get home immediately he started to feel the urge. Sometimes he got antsy when watching TV or in the

Smoke Room. It was then that I had to do my best de-escalation work. For some reason, once he was better, Terry liked me.

I sat next to him in the Smoke Room one evening.

'Jim,' he said, 'I'm gaun hame.'

'Yeah,' I answered, a familiar sinking feeling in my gut. 'Won't be long now. You're doing really well.'

'Naw, I mean I'm gaun hame now.'

'Cannae do it, pal. You've got to wait till Dr Bankstreet gives the green light.'

'If I don't get hame the night, I'm gonnae go right ahead.'

'That would be a pity, man. Dr Bankstreet is talkin' about you gettin' escorted time out tomorrow. Next day at the latest. That's the start of the process. Home soon after that.'

'Bankstreet? What gives that cow the right to decide mah fate?'

'Her degree in psychiatry and her seniority in the service?' I risked.

He looked at me, cigarette smoke curling in a warning way from the side of his mouth.

'Jim, you takin' the piss here?'

'Perish the thought, Tel. No me. Just answering your question. That's what lets Dr Bankstreet decide these things.'

'But it's mah life we're talkin' about here.'

'Sure. But think about this. Whether you like her or no – and I can see why you might resent her – she's trying to do the best for you and your life. She doesnae want to see you back in a place like this. It's like sending somebody home when they've still got an infection or something. They have to come back in. Nobody wants that for you, pal.'

He chewed this for a moment.

'She better get her finger out her arse then, Jim.'

'Oh she is,' I assured him. 'If you listen carefully, you can hear the pop . . .' I flicked my finger out my cheek '. . . as she does.'

He laughed.

'Right, Jim. Whatever you say.'

29

Demoniac frenzy, moping melancholy
And moon-struck madness.
John Milton, *Paradise Lost*

Terry got home fairly quickly, but that was a time I tend to associate with increased tension on the ward and a higher incidence of violence and restraint than was customary. Several patients who had been on the ward for a long time were discharged together, and they all seemed to be the quieter, less aggressive or demanding ones: Theo, Stannie, Voytek and people of that kidney. At the same time two or three people were admitted within a few days of each other who were suspicious and hostile, and that made for a combustible mixture on the floor. I subscribed to Charlie's dictum of unconditional nursing wholeheartedly, but I'm a human being with human character flaws. This was four or five years into my time on 25. I found it hard to feel too much sympathy for a man who was trying to kick the jaw off my face, or a woman who was prepared to throw a mug of hot coffee in the face of another staff member.

I'd never had any issue with taking part in restraints. Although like everyone else I'd rather they hadn't been necessary, I had to admit that at times they were. If I was present, I participated. The other guys were strong, quick and skilful. I only helped out. I had no illusions about my part in the process. The perennial bum man. Occasionally

I took a blow, as in the grapple with Bryce, and I was prepared to accept that. I certainly didn't want, however, to *keep* taking blows. The set-up on the ward at that time suggested this might happen more often. And, by then, I'd become a grandfather for the first time. If they were to make a movie of my life, this is the point at which the actor playing me (George Clooney, for preference, playing against type) would stub out his fag and growl, 'I'm getting too old for this shit.'

The first admission wasn't too aggressive – at least not on the floor of 25. An old lag called Sniff, he had been admitted after an altercation with a fellow patient in 24, during the course of which he had dug a deep furrow in the other man's face with a sharpened plastic protractor.

Sniff was in his sixties and had, as a much younger man, done time in Barlinnie for the attempted murder by stabbing of his brother. Now he cast yearning glances back at what he saw as the most meaningful time of his life: as a convict in the Bar-L. That was ineffably sad. But he mitigated this by writing about it. He wrote his memoirs on sheets of green foolscap paper that he had obviously liberated from some institution – maybe even the hoosegow itself – at some time in his past. He wrote in a large, cursive script in pencil, relating tales of the people and incidents he had known there, including the famous Jimmy Boyle. Once he found out that I was an English graduate and interested in writing myself, he came and asked if I'd be good enough to read them for him. I assented and often passed the time by immersing myself in Sniff's memoirs. They were very good – thrilling and amusing by turns – written in a swift and pacy style. I told him I thought they were excellent and that he should consider trying to have them published. He looked appalled at the thought.

'Oh no,' he said earnestly. 'There are people who would seek wevenge if they wed anything I'd witten about them.'

I let it lie.

I found Sniff an attractive character, despite the assault with the protractor and rumours of previous attacks using sharp weapons. He was tall and elegant, with a wicked sense of humour and a speech impediment that reminded me very much of John Sweeney, the bus driver I'd nursed years ago in the old asylum. He liked to pass the time of day with me when he had a moment from his busy writing schedule, say at coffee time or smoko.

'Why do they call you Sniff?' I asked him.

'Because my name's Smith,' he said. 'And my nickname awose fwom a childish inability to pwonounce it. Other kids' inability, I mean. I could always pwonounce it pehfectly. One of the few things I could pwonounce.'

'They say you cut Freddie with a protractor.'

'Pehfectly cowwect.'

'Why did you have a protractor?'

'Because I'm vewy intewested in geometwy,' he answered with a smile. 'You never know when you might need to measure an angle accuwately.'

'What was it about?'

'Well, I wike to photogwaph women's bottoms, and he found a photogwaph I'd taken of a female he's wather fond of—'

'Woah, okay. Sorry I asked.'

I found his sense of humour irresistible. One Sunday morning at coffee time Sniff was at the hatch and the

Dayroom TV was showing a service to mark the sixtieth anniversary of the D-Day landings. While I poured his coffee and passed him the biscuit box, he stood with his face averted, watching the programme. Then he turned as I handed him his drink.

'Sixtieth annivessawy of D-Day,' he commented.

'Aye.'

'Bwing back any memowies?' he asked with an impish grin and sidled off, chuckling.

Sniff was something of a pocket philosopher. Every morning, when he emerged from his room at the top of the bedded area to walk down to breakfast, he would have some bon mot, some *pensée*, to share with me. I suspect he spent an enjoyable hour or so the night before, thinking them up.

'If Adam and Eve had thwee sons, as it says in the Bible, where did the west of the human wace come fwom?' he asked one morning.

'Would an academic textbook on the histowy of circumcision need to start with a pwepuce? Ha ha ha,' was another day's poser.

My personal favourite was: 'Who told Johnny Cash he could sing?'

It was the Sniff equivalent of Thought for the Day.

I asked him once about the attempted murder of his brother and why he had done it. He paused and looked at me with his knowing little smile.

'You know, Dennis,' he said, 'there's nothing quite like the sensation of a blade passing thwough human tissue. Take my word fow it.'

I did.

* * *

The following Friday, around afternoon coffee time, a male patient was brought to us by the police. Luke and I were the only two males on duty at the time. Charlie was on holiday; Clyde had gone on a half-day, Gordon and John were on their lunch hour. There were three policemen accompanying the patient.

Robbie was from the city, a paranoid schizophrenic who was known to psychiatric services there and had presented no management problems up to that time. He had ceased complying with medication some weeks previously, and there had been a conspicuous deterioration despite several interventions by medical staff. All attempts to get him back on his meds had failed. His consultant had tried to get him to come into hospital in a final bid to restart his course, but he had become extremely aggressive when the doctor and two male nurses had gone to his flat. A quick call to Dr Bankstreet had elicited her assent to his admission to the Locked Ward.

Now, as I looked at Robbie, standing between two policemen in his handcuffs, I thought that we wouldn't be discussing too much literature together. He stood and regarded each of us in turn with a look of cold and implacable contempt. When he looked at me, my sphincter puckered so far into itself that, if I'd stuck a straw up it, I could have emptied a pail of dandelion and burdock via the back door. This man meant business.

Geraldine explained to him that he would have to receive some medication. She would prefer that he take it orally but, if he refused, she was perfectly ready to give him it by injection.

'Naw,' he said. 'Nae drugs.'

'I'm sorry, but our consultant has prescribed that you should take these. You have no choice, since you're

259

sectioned under the Mental Health Act. Your only choice is whether to take the tablets or get a jag.'

'Anybody jags me is going to regret it.'

This was a script we'd read before.

'Want us to keep the cuffs on him till you give him it?' asked one of the policemen.

'Yeah,' said Geraldine with a sigh, turning to go. 'Since he seems determined to get it that way. Can you stay till I do it?'

'Aye, but not too much longer.'

'Five minutes,' said Geraldine and left to draw it up.

'YOU'RE NO GIVIN' ME ANY A THAT POISON!'

His sudden, throat-ripping yell had me halfway up the curtains, like a cat. It was obvious that he was as frightened as I was. Only he was frightened of the situation and what drugs Geraldine might be injecting into him. I was just frightened of what he was going to do.

'Hang on a minute, Den,' said Luke. 'Back in a jiffy.'

Where the fuck was he going? He was gone. Now there was me, three policemen and Robbie. If the police uncuffed him, he would have me pinging off the walls like a squash ball. I could see the next day's headlines all too clearly in my mind's eye:

MEEK HIPPY GRANDAD KILLED AT WORK
Devout Coward Slain By Madman
Garotted With His Own Underpants

'Where'd your mate say he was going?' one of the Bow Street Runners asked me. His tone of voice made it clear that he considered Luke's absence gross dereliction of duty and the whole thing probably my fault.

'No idea.'

He looked at me disdainfully.

'Said he'd be back in a jiffy,' observed one of his mates wryly.

'Aye. He said that.'

I wasn't concerned about Luke being back in a jiffy so much as not wanting to go out of there in a jiffy *bag*. Then he returned.

'Ronnie and Tosh are comin' over from 24. Just got Rona to phone them over.'

I could have kissed him. By the time Geraldine returned with her needles and other paraphernalia in a stainless-steel kidney dish, her hands in blue disposable gloves, Ronnie and Tosh were with us.

'Okay,' said Geraldine. 'Place him on the bed, face down.'

'DON'T GIVE ME POISON! NO DRUGS!'

The policemen lowered him by the shoulders and he lay on his stomach, his head turned to the side so that he could not see what Geraldine was doing.

'Your faces are all noted,' he rasped. 'You'll pay for this.'

Geraldine went through the procedure, tugging his jeans down, cleaning the area with an antiseptic wipe before injecting him twice. She cleaned the spot again, patted on a sticking plaster and tugged his jeans back up before leaving. Robbie had made no sound at all during the actual injection. Nor did he now, as John appeared back from lunch.

'Just brought in,' said Luke.

'Pam told me,' said John.

'Kosher to take these cuffs off now?' asked a policeman.

'Aye,' said Luke. 'There's enough of us here now.'

'He's quiet enough, like,' said Gordon, now appearing.

'Sit up,' said the cop.

Robbie rolled over and sat up. The policeman unlocked his handcuffs. Immediately Robbie's right leg shot up from the edge of the bed. Gordon was unfortunate enough – or gormless enough – to be standing directly in front of him. Robbie's foot connected solidly with his groin and Gordon went down like a bookie's line. At the same time Robbie shot up from the bed, smacked his right fist into Tosh's cheek and felled him. One of the coppers grabbed him round the neck and got an elbow in the solar plexus for his pains. He clung on grimly, though. Then all of us – except Gordon, who was rolling around the floor in agony – leaped in: three policemen, John, Luke, Ronnie, Tosh – who had got up from the floor again – and me. Eight people. Robbie stopped, staggered and began to revolve slowly, trying to shake us loose. Geraldine and Rona came running in. Someone had set off the alarm.

'What can we do?' asked Geraldine.

'Treble Three,' shouted Luke.

'And get Gordon out. He's taken a nut shot,' said John.

Geraldine jerked her thumb for Rona to run and send out a Treble Three. She then bent down and eased Gordon into a sitting position.

'Stand up,' she urged.

'Can't.'

'You can. Here, I'll help you up. Treatment Room for you.'

Gordon hirpled out, Geraldine's arm around his shoulders. Meanwhile, Robbie was blundering about the room, half sagging to his knees and yet, somehow, from somewhere, finding the strength to almost stand upright and move a few paces. He was straining till the blood vessels stood out on his forehead, his neck muscles taut like wires, his breath a rasping croak.

Pounding feet. Two porters and a male nurse from the elderly ward. They sprang into the fray. It took the eleven of us, hanging off him like ticks, to bring him down. Eventually, sheer physical effort combined with the effects of the medication did the trick. One by one we disengaged and he fell onto the bed sideways.

'That's one strong bastard,' said one of the policemen admiringly.

'I'll get you. I'll get. You. All,' said Robbie, slurring through exhaustion. And then he was asleep.

The policemen left. The reinforcements left, except for Ronnie, who had permission to stay and make up our numbers. Luke hefted Robbie's holdall onto his table and opened it to start checking his gear. He gave a low whistle.

'Have a fuckin' look at this,' he said.

In the holdall were three thin metal files sharpened to bayonet standard, a hunting knife, a cut-throat razor with a black plastic handle and two golf balls with nails driven through them. They looked like old naval mines and were probably just as lethal.

'Good job he didn't get to use any of this shit,' said Luke through gritted teeth. 'I take it the polis didnae check his bag when he packed.'

'You cannae putt with balls like that,' I said.

'Bet Gordon's are like that the now,' said Ronnie.

Geraldine came in.

'Look at this,' said Luke.

'Write it all down,' she said, 'and then get them locked away safely.'

'How's Gordon?'

'Sitting in the Treatment Room with his feet up and his legs splayed. An ice pack on the affected area.'

'You mean you didnae kiss it all better for him?' John smiled. Then didn't smile. 'Only joking, Gerry.'

'You can stop joking. Get that stuff away. Two men on special. The rest of you out and get the ward back to normal. Coffee would be a good idea.'

Robbie slept through the rest of the shift, probably because of the enormous physical strain he had gone through, but also because of the drugs after such a long period of abstinence. Our shift had the long weekend off after that. When we came back on the Tuesday the handover informed us that Robbie had been restrained and medicated twice more over the intervening period, but also that they had worked out a modus vivendi. For myself, so long as there was the prospect of vivendi without any hassle, I'd settle for any modus.

Robbie remained extremely reserved and suspicious around male staff. He was, however, willing to work with female colleagues. It may have been a testosterone thing, a throwback to our days in the trees, seeing any other male as a threat, or it may have been simply that he was used to female family members, such as his mother and sisters. Whatever the reason, we were happy to go along with his wishes. Rona or Ursula would wake him in the morning and inform him that breakfast was being served in the Executive Lounge at that moment. Pamela or Geraldine would give him his meds. He was still unhappy about having to take them, but he agreed to, so long as he could see the names on the bottles and blister packs, see the girls popping the pills out of the pack or pouring the syrup into the little plastic medicine cup, and receive them from their hands only.

He would sit in the top corner of the Dayroom, well away from other patients. He always wore his soft leather jacket and a checked shirt. If a male member of staff came in, he would regard him distrustfully. He was not much better with male patients but few bothered him. If we needed to speak to him or have him do something, it was always one of the girls who asked him. Even when it came to coffee time, if I was on the hatch when the patients were queuing up for their cuppa, I could see Robbie eyeing me balefully. If I called to him, 'Something to drink, Robbie?' he'd turn his nose up and look away. Maybe snarl, 'Naw.' One of the girls could get him to drink something and have a biscuit, but even then, like so many others, he'd insist on watching every move they made before accepting the drink.

The first time Dr Bankstreet interviewed him was enlightening. When Pamela asked him to go into the Interview Room with the doctor, he point-blank refused. Dr Bankstreet sought him out in the Dayroom and asked him personally if he would agree to be interviewed. He looked at her, looked her over thoroughly, obviously decided that this was not a man dressed up, and agreed sullenly. Pamela sat in on the interview. That was normally done by at least one of us blokes, but the difficulties in this case were obvious. Nonetheless, when Pamela closed the door, John, Luke and I hung about in the corridor outside as backup. Out-of-sight backup. Like the Temptations.

Over the ensuing weeks Robbie became gradually less aggressive but hardly any less suspicious of the male staff – in particular, me. The time came for his escorted walks around the grounds and to the filling station. As custom dictated, he went with Charlie first. Then with John. Then with Luke. Came the day it was my turn to do the escort. I found Robbie in his favoured seat by the Dayroom window.

'I'm going out to the garage, Robbie,' I said. 'Do you want anything? Want to come with me for the walk?'

He shook his head.

'Look, buddy,' I said. 'I know you're not sure of me, but I'm the one who's going out to the garage. If you don't come with me, I'm not sure if there'll be another chance today.'

He looked at me as if he'd just turned me up on the sole of his shoe.

'Happy for you to come,' I said, and shrugged as non-committally as I could. He had to feel the decision was his alone.

'Wait a minute till I get my money?' he mumbled.

'Sure.'

We walked in silence. I'd tried one or two harmless conversational openers but he'd blanked everything. I waited at the back of the filling-station shop while he made his purchases – the staff knew all us orderlies by sight. Then, on the way back, he stopped for a moment to light a cigarette. I dallied while he turned his back to the wind. Then I fell back into step with him, wondering when the 'dilly' part of 'dilly-dally' fell out of use. My mother had used it when I was a child. As in the old music-hall lyric: 'And don't dilly-dally on the way.' She'd often warned me not to dilly-dally. And here I was now, never to dilly-dally again. Dally, yes, but dilly, no. Although I have been known from time to time to shilly-shally. But that's a story for another time. These were the fine thoughts exercising my mind at that moment.

'I remember you,' he said, none too friendly. 'Don't think I don't.'

'Remember me?' I said. 'From where?'

'That union meeting in town. I remember you, all right. You're a married man. You wear a wedding ring. And you went away with that woman delegate from Newcastle.'

'Did I?' I said. 'I wonder if I got anywhere with her.'

'Don't try and be smart,' he said. 'I remember that. I was disgusted.'

'You're making a mistake, Robbie,' I said. 'I've never been with a Newcastle trade union delegate in my life. What union are you talking about, anyway?'

'Transport and General. You know.'

'Never been a member of the T and G, old son. Nor had a dalliance with a Geordie delegate.'

His lip curled so far it disappeared up his left nostril.

'You say,' he said.

And we discussed the matter no further. For the rest of his time with us he treated me with ill-disguised contempt for my imaginary infidelity with an unknown lady from Newcastle. I wonder who she was and who it was who actually did enjoy her favours. Another man with the rare combination of poetic soul and gently sardonic wit that I possess, obviously.

30

That wench is stark mad or wonderful froward.
William Shakespeare, *The Taming of the Shrew*

Elaine came back at this time. The girl who had given me the shark look on my first day was readmitted. After that first day she hadn't remained long in the ward. At the time she was only seventeen, and the Locked Ward was not considered the most appropriate place for a girl of that age. Dr Bankstreet had found her a place in a specialist adolescent unit, and she was transferred there. Now she was back, in her twenties and considerably more dangerous. She had acquired a taste for opiates in the intervening years and was then on a methadone programme.

Methadone is a heroin substitute. The thinking behind giving addicts regular doses of methadone is that it does away with the illegal drug, reduces crime associated with heroin addiction, allows addicts (slowly) to get healthier and reduces the incidence of diseases like hepatitis and HIV that are commonly transmitted through infected needles. Methadone works by satisfying the addict's craving for the drug without producing the undesirable aspects. (Although recent research has suggested that some people on methadone programmes are just as likely to commit crime and take heroin as any other drug addict.)

It is what is called a 'controlled' drug. The use of such drugs is licensed under certain conditions in medical contexts. The drugs have to be securely stored in a double-locked steel safety cabinet fixed to a wall and issue has to be recorded in ink in a bound register. On Ward 25 two trained nurses had to countersign the issue of methadone to any patient.

At certain meds times Elaine would be called into the Treament Room and handed a small plastic cup containing a measure of thick green syrup rather like Fairy Liquid. This was her methadone, and she put it away with urgent enjoyment, turning the cup and squeezing the plastic to extract all the syrup she could. She would be extremely fractious of a morning till she got her methadone. If she felt it was not coming quickly enough, she would slam her door against the wall and loudly demand her medication.

'Mah med-eyes!' she would roar at the air. 'Ah wahnt mah fuckin' med-eyes!'

This was a piece of cant she had picked up in a women's prison. She had been sent there a few years previously for threatening an infant in a pram with a broken bottle, as a means of extorting from its terrified young mother the price of another high. In prison she had acquired several other unpleasant attributes, including a tendency to explosive violence and complete sexual shamelessness. I hesitate to call it sexual disinhibition, because it wasn't quite what Lesley had had. Elaine just took sexual gratification where she could, and when she felt inclined. It was part of her utter contempt for other people.

She had first got in trouble through an obsession she had developed for a female social worker. Let me state here that I don't think that Elaine was gay, because gayness suggests

269

love for a person of the same gender. Love was not an emotion that, to my mind, Elaine ever experienced. Not for anyone else, certainly. Caring for someone else, their feelings, their happiness? Not Elaine. But her social worker was dedicated, diligent, professional and thorough. She spent a lot of time helping Elaine when she came out of the adolescent unit, and, consequently, Elaine got hung up on her. At this distance of time, I can't recall anything about Elaine's home background except that she hated her mother, so I assume she hadn't grown up in *The Little House on the Prairie*. Perhaps the experience of another adult human caring for her in some positive way was entirely new to her.

In any case, Elaine got the hots for this woman. She was infatuated, and infatuated bad. She told her one day, when she visited Elaine at her flat, that she loved her and wanted to go to bed with her. Then. Right there and then.

The social worker did not feel the same way at all. Nor anything remotely like it. Very calmly but very plainly she told Elaine that she felt no attraction to her in that sense, nor ever could. She was happily in love with someone else. It was best that Elaine forget the whole thing. She didn't mean to hurt her feelings in any way, but it was not possible for anything to happen between them.

Elaine threw a strop that was Ancient Greek in its scope and intensity, and threatened the social worker with the direst consequences if she did not humour her. The woman, sensing that this was not going well, managed somehow to extricate herself from the situation, and the flat, and made fairly good speed away from there. When she got back to the office, she spoke to her line manager and made it clear that she could not continue to be responsible for Elaine's case, for the reasons outlined above. And she was removed from it, a man being appointed to Elaine's care in her place.

Elaine was remorseless. She phoned the woman night and day, both her landline and mobile numbers. She wrote three letters every day. She took to hanging about outside the woman's house and office. When she was served with an injunction restraining her from going within several hundred yards of either location, Elaine went to the social worker's front door on a Saturday morning. She knocked loudly on it. When the woman answered, she found Elaine with her jeans and knickers lowered to her ankles, squatting and pissing like a Blackpool donkey on her doorstep. Elaine adjusted her clothes and, with a final disdainful toss of the head, walked down the path and out into the street. That cost her her first spell in custody.

I'll put my cards on the table here. I found Elaine a very hard person to like. In fact, I didn't like her at all. Over the years several patients were difficult to strike up a relationship with. Others were, as I've said, hard to like. It was the same as any other walk of life or place of work. Most people are easy to get on with or at least tolerate. Some are harder. Some you wouldn't nod to in the desert. Some you wouldn't piss on if they were on fire. So it was in the ward, and why should it be any different? My whole thesis is that we shouldn't expect people with mental disorders to be too different from anyone else.

For her first few days on this admission, staff kept an eye on her from a discreet remove until her behaviour dictated otherwise. Her shamelessness was the first cause for concern. She would go to the loo with both doors open – bedroom door and lavatory door – so that it was not too difficult for anyone passing in the corridor to see her passing in the lavatory. Pamela gave her a bollocking for that, but Elaine only sneered. One night about midnight a female member of the night staff found her lying on her bed, enjoying some solitary pleasure with the light on. She was reprimanded very roundly for that. The very next night about the same time, when staff went to check the Smoke Room as they closed things down for the night, Elaine was found there in a rather advanced state of undress and performing what the papers love to call a 'sex act' with a male patient. She was put on close with one female nurse.

This lasted a week until she gave her word to Charlie and the chief night nurse that she wouldn't be quite so brazen in her pursuit of sexual gratification. For a few days all went well, but then they became rapidly worse.

Also on the ward then was a young woman called Sadie. Sadie was extremely striking in appearance: tall, slim, with exquisitely fine features. Her eyes were large and elfin. Her cheeks were high. Her lips were full and slightly down turned. Her hair curled delicately around the nape of her neck. She had, besides, an air of dreamy remoteness that added to her strange and slightly transcendental beauty. She looked vaguely unreal, as if she was being dreamed by a seahorse.

But, tragically, she suffered from a degenerative disorder of the brain. This was a horrible illness that caused her, in moments of extreme anguish, to shriek for minutes at a time in the most blood-curdling way. Charlie theorised that she did this because she was aware of the nature of her condition and of the horrors that lay ahead of her. Luke commented once that anyone passing the ward when Sadie was screaming like that would go away with an image of the ward as being like the old asylums, where lunatics howled down long, dimly lit corridors. It was agonising to hear. Usually Sadie did this in her room, but one day she did it in the Dayroom.

Elaine was off close. Sadie materialised out of her room and quietly passed down the corridor of the bedded area, past the Nurses' Station and into the Dayroom. Luke, Rona, Ursula and I were seated around the Station, shooting the breeze. It was a moment of calm. Elaine came out of her room and gave her usual smart-arsed smirk when she saw us.

'Gonnae gie us a smoke, man?' she asked me.

'No.'

'How no?'

'Because I don't have enough for myself for the rest of the shift. So I can't give you one.'

'Baldy bastard!' she spat at me.

'So am I,' I said.

'Gonnae gie us a smoke, man?' she asked Luke.

'No. For the same reason.'

'Fuck youse, man. Heh, Rona . . .'

'I don't smoke, Elaine.'

'Neither do I,' added Ursula.

'Fuck this!' she shouted.

And then Sadie's anguished screaming tore the air between the Dayroom and us. This was unusual. It irked Elaine beyond telling.

'There's that mad bitch screamin' again! Why the fuck do youse let her dae it?'

'Because she's unwell,' said Rona.

'Bad enough when she's in her room. It's ten times worse oot here.'

'Yeah, well, like Rona said, the lassie's no well.'

Elaine paced and fumed for ten or twenty seconds.

'That din is daein' mah heid in!' she yelped and stalked away. I assumed she was off to the Smoke Room to try and cadge a wheeze from a fellow patient. But suddenly there was the dull thump of a fist on flesh and a quite different cry from Sadie, a sharp cry of physical pain. Elaine stalked back into the night area.

'That stupit bitch's fell against the door,' she said and slammed her own door shut.

Rona and I ran into the Dayroom. Sadie was slumped on the floor. She was holding the right side of her face and crying. She was evidently hurt.

'What happened, Sadie?' said Rona.

But Sadie didn't answer. She seldom spoke, except to answer yes or no on occasions.

'Take your hand, away, Sadie,' I said as Rona gently removed it. Her cheek was swelling and bruising almost visibly.

'That bad bism's hit her,' said Rona. 'Sadie, did Elaine hit you?'

'Did anybody hit you?' I asked at the same time.

Sadie cried.

'Is it sore?' asked Rona.

'Yes,' Sadie whimpered.

Geraldine appeared.

'What's going on here?' She sounded like Edna May Oliver playing a 1930s headmistress.

'Sadie was in here and started screaming. Elaine mumped about the noise doing her head in and marched through. There was a thump and Sadie yelled. Then Elaine came back through, said Sadie had hit her face off the door and went to her room. Dennis and I came through and found Sadie like this.'

Geraldine took one look at Sadie's face.

'Take her to the Treatment Room, Rona. I'll be through in a minute. Dennis, phone the duty doc.'

And Geraldine strode off to interview Elaine. She put her back on close. Male or female staff. Luke got the first watch.

The duty doc duly came. Sadie had a depressed fracture of the cheekbone. It was the doctor's opinion that the injury had been sustained as the result of a blow from a fist rather than from an impersonal object like a door.

'That's a bad fuckin' bitch,' opined Gordon.

From then on Elaine became less and less open to reason. She erupted into squalls of bad temper. She shouted abuse at staff and patients. She took particular exception to Geraldine. One afternoon Geraldine was dealing with the drinks and snacks at three o'clock. Elaine came through with Clyde in tow as her close observer, walked straight to the front of the hatch and barked at Geraldine, 'Coffee. Three sugars and milk.'

'End of the queue, Elaine,' said Geraldine, 'and wait your turn. There are three in front of you.'

'Fuck them,' said Elaine. 'Coffee, three sugars and milk.'

'Come on, Elaine. Wait your turn,' said Clyde quietly.

'Fuck that bitch. She's only pissin' me around.'

'Come on, Elaine,' said Clyde, taking her by the arm.

'Get off me, you bastard!'

'Elaine!' snapped Geraldine.

Elaine snatched the coffee from the front girl at the hatch and launched it at Geraldine. Fortunately, Geraldine guessed what was coming and ducked before the liquid could do her any damage. It's an old lag's trick, scalding coffee with plenty of sugar thrown in someone's face. The sugar makes it stick to the skin.

Clyde grabbed Elaine – seriously now – and set off his alarm. By the time Geraldine got round from the pantry, and Luke and I had raced into the Dayroom, Elaine had landed one or two heavy blows on Clyde's face. Geraldine, Luke and I hauled her off him, but she struggled and fought, dug the heel of her shoe into Geraldine's instep, spat at Luke, and tried to knee me in the family jewels. We half dragged, half frogmarched her through to her room and put her into restraint on the bed. Geraldine drew up two blues and a larry and sedated her.

Thereafter, she was restricted to her room except for meals and specialed by two at all times, two males preferably. One day she tried to barge her way past John and me, but we put her back in the room. Four times she tried it.

'Do it once more, and you'll be jagged.'

'FUCK YOUSE! YA FUCKIN' POOFS! FUCK YOUSE ALL! AH'LL GET THAT HOOR, SEE IF I DON'T!'

Then she grabbed the door and slammed it shut, trying to catch John with it.

'She's a wee Christmas bell, isn't she?' I said.

In fact, horribly, she tried the same trick during the night shift and severed the top of a female nurse's finger. Those doors were heavy, with a metal strike plate. It must have been an agonising injury. I promise you, my skin crawls as I write this. Moves were set in train to transfer Elaine to a secure unit in the city.

And then came her *pièce de résistance*.

It was lunchtime. I was passing out the trays, and Geraldine was walking around the dining area. John and

Luke brought Elaine in and sat her at a table on her own. Geraldine came over to the hatch and collected Elaine's meal. She took it over to her table and set the tray down before her. As Elaine removed the metal lids from her dishes, Geraldine paused to pass the time of day with some of the guys. Elaine whisked the detached section of her menu from the tray and onto the table. It slid along the formica and was about to fall off the edge when Geraldine stopped it with her right hand flat on the table.

'Careful, Elaine,' she admonished.

And, in a blink, Elaine stuck her fork into the back of Geraldine's hand. Just like that. The quickness of the hand deceives the eye. The tines of the fork were half buried in Geraldine's hand. There is little flesh on the back of the hand, so that gives you some idea of the force with which Elaine had rammed the fork into her. Geraldine screamed. The guys ripped Elaine out of her seat and bundled her through to her room. I answered the alarm and we got her restrained. She hissed, 'Told you I'd get the hoor.'

She went to the Big Hoose three days later. Nobody missed her.

31

We have but two sorts of people in the house, and both under the whip,
that's fools and madmen; the one has not wit enough to be knaves,
and the other not knavery enough to be fools.

Thomas Middleton and William Rowley, _The Changeling_

Next on the Most Wanted list came Barry. He was known to the team who had worked in the asylum, but had not been admitted to the Locked Ward in the hospital before this presentation. He more or less self-admitted. He pitched up at the ward door one Saturday morning, alone. When John spoke to him through the squawk box, he said he needed to talk to Dr Bankstreet right away because he hadn't been taking his meds and knew he was unwell, really unwell, as a consequence. Charlie wasn't on that day, so Geraldine told John to let Barry in till she spoke to him.

'Who is it?' I asked John as he pressed the door release and rose to open the Buffer Zone door.

'Barry,' he said. 'Long-lost sparring partner of mine.'

When he came in, Barry looked ill, no doubt about it. He was gaunt and haggard, his complexion a horrid greyish-yellow, and his eyes standing out, in John's expression, 'like a whippet's nuts'. There was a perceptible tremor to his limbs when he stood or sat. Geraldine got him to sit in the Smoke Room until she could speak to the SHO on duty that weekend. John and I hung about outside the Smoke Room and cast an occasional glance at him through the

Judas window. He was smoking chains. Sometimes he lifted his head as if someone had called him and looked at nothing. I nudged John and pointed it out.

'Hallucinating.'

'Maybe. He's a cute bastard and he might be faking it.'

'Alas,' I said, 'how is it with you that you do bend your eye on vacancy, and with the incorporal air do hold discourse?'

John looked at me as if I were dafter than Barry.

'I swear to God, wee man,' he said, 'sometimes you talk the most unadulterated pish.'

'Pish? That's Shakespeare! Hamlet! Hamlet, Prince of Pish.'

'They're needin' to give you a bed, pal.'

'What did you mean when you said he might be faking it?'

'Just that. Barry's a shrewd customer. He's here for a reason. When did you ever hear of a patient wanting to get *in*to Ward 25? They're all desperate to get *out* of it. Mention the ward to them outside and they usually run like three blind mice. He's here because for some reason this is the safest place for him to be. He's on the run from somethin'.'

'But he's hallucinating,' I said.

'Barry's an old hand,' John said, shaking his head. 'He knows how to act mad. He needs a bolthole for some reason and this is it.'

Barry was admitted despite John's reservations. The SHO diagnosed a relapse of his paranoid schizophrenia. That evening we heard reports of a near-fatal stabbing that had taken place in a local village the night before. This had happened at a drinking session in the house of another person known to psychiatric services. The injured man

279

was in intensive care up the stairs. No one questioned at the scene was admitting that they knew anything about the incident. The agreed tale seemed to be that the victim had gone outside and been attacked by unknown hands.

'Pish,' said John pithily. Or maybe it was 'Pith' he said pishily. One or the other. His meaning was clear, whatever he said. 'If it wasnae Barry that plunged the guy, Barry at least knows who dunnit and why.'

'Certainly,' agreed Luke. 'Barry wouldn't hesitate. He is the kind of geezer who gets the red mist descending and then, when it lifts again, somebody's lying awfu' hurt, awfu' close to Barry.'

The next day, Sunday, another man was admitted. Not for us in 25 the long lie, the full English and the Sunday papers before a quiet pint and a preprandial dose in the armchair. No, no. Full on, 24/7. The cutting edge. The task force. The shock troops. Simon was admitted – admitted by dragging – from 24, where he had gone apeshit over someone changing the TV channel without consulting him. Such trivia are often the triggers for aggression. And not only in psychie wards.

The alarms went off, and a rapid scan of the board showed that the problem was in 24. A quick look through the long window in the main door showed us someone in the long window of *their* main door beckoning furiously. John, Luke and I went over. There were only two men on duty in 24, and they were having the devil's own job managing Simon. We huckled him over to 25, pushing, pulling, lifting and propelling in various other ways as he struggled, swore and eventually dug his heels into the floor.

This made a fine squeaking noise as we hauled him over the road to the IPCU.

Geraldine was already in the Treatment Room, drawing one up. John and Luke held him pinioned by the arms. I stood by, trying to look like I could unleash all sorts of shit if he started messing.

'Right, Simon,' said Geraldine, approaching with her works in a kidney dish. 'Drop your trousers, please.'

'Oh aye,' said Simon suspiciously. 'What's all this about?'

'Just drop your trousers,' advised John. 'You're getting a jag.'

Simon stepped away from them and dropped his trousers and pants, so that he was naked to the socks. 'In the arse or in the prick?' he said.

'Just in the buttock,' said Geraldine coolly. 'You can pull your underpants back up.'

'Right,' said Simon, doing so. 'I thought this was some sort of bum bandits' day out. Gang of homos standing around, watching some other guy getting it up the arse.'

We were well used to this sort of talk. Nobody commented on Simon's little outburst; we just watched Geraldine professionally and skilfully administer the injection.

'Right, Simon. You can dress yourself again, and the boys will show you to your room.'

We showed him into one of the rooms on the courtyard side and he said, 'Aye, okay,' and then lay on the top of his bed and fell asleep.

His notes were enlightening. He had a history of torturing and killing birds and small animals. Impaling them on spikes. Clubbing them to death. Setting fire to them. These were a few of his favourite things. Which is bad

281

enough in itself, beyond doubt. Sadistic and brutal. But the literature suggests that such behaviour is often a precursor to sensationally more serious activity.

'That's a sign of a serial killer, I'm sure,' said Luke as we sat around the table at dinner that evening.

'What is?' asked Ursula.

'Torturing animals. Your serial killer often starts that way. Form of control.'

'Psycho killer, *qu'est-ce que c'est?*' said Gordon. Nobody paid him any attention.

'Is that true?' Ursula looked at Charlie, who sighed.

'Sometimes. Sometimes. But there's a whole raft of other indicators,' said Charlie, forking rice and Thai green curry into his mouth.

'Like what?' said John.

'Och, a number of things. There's often a history of physical abuse . . .'

'Not mentioned in the notes.'

'. . . mother's boy syndrome . . .'

'Check.'

'. . . anti-social tendencies in adolescence . . .'

'Check.'

'. . . an interest in pyromania . . .'

'Check!' said Luke. 'Fuck. We've got Jack the Ripper Junior here! Son of Jack!'

'Not funny, Luke, and hardly likely,' said Geraldine.

Charlie nodded. 'But a man worth watching all the same.'

Actually, Simon kept himself very much to himself over the next short while. He had a friend, an older man with a slight smack of having slept in a cardboard box about him. This man visited several times and brought a small travelling chessboard. They would set this up at a

Dayroom table and castle the king, or twiddle the bishop, for most of visiting time. This man must also have brought Simon's music collection with him at some point, or even at various ones. One afternoon I had occasion to call upon Simon in his room, and he had set up his CDs in a series of ranks along the window sill.

'Sizeable collection,' I said.

'Aye.'

And it was an impressive one, at least to an old hippy and child of the '60s. I scanned the serried spines. Which is not a thing I often get the chance to do. (Well, when was the last time *you* scanned serried spines?) The Beatles, the Stones, the Kinks, the Doors, the Grateful Dead, Led Zeppelin, Free and other artists that I had revered in my youth, were all represented. Mind you, so also were Yes, Wishbone Ash and sundry other wankery that I would never have tolerated on a turntable in them thar days. I would rather have melted their LPs over a candle and made plant-pot holders of them. Pink Floyd I would have allowed only when the chief elf and acid casualty, Syd Barrett himself, was with them. Other stuff that I could take or leave, such as Slade and the Nice, was also in there. It was an astonishingly eclectic assortment.

'Good stuff too, most of it,' I said (rather patronisingly, I now realise).

'Yeah. I pick it up cheap at markets.'

'You've got good taste, Simon.'

'You mean it agrees with yours?' he said. 'That's what folk usually mean when they say things like that.'

'Okay, smart-arse.'

(Some months later, Simon was temporarily granted the tenancy of a flat in a local village. Unfortunately he took ill again, and John, Clyde and I were dispatched to fetch him. The floor of his little living room was carpeted, wall to wall, with what looked like glass powder or glass snow and sounded like it too as it crunched underfoot.

'What the hell's this' asked John.

'CDs,' said Simon.

The entire astonishingly eclectic assortment had been broken, then splintered, then pulverised.

'What'd you do that for?' I asked him.

'Got fed up with them. I'm into Abba now.'

Simon had a penchant at this time for having an evening shower around seven o'clock and then spending the last hour and a half of our dayshift watching TV or playing pool in his pyjamas. But his were not the old-fashioned winceyette jim-jams in deckchair stripes so dear to the days of my youth. Simon's 'sleepwear', as he insisted on calling it, was in navy and consisted of a round-necked T-shirt with short sleeves and a pair of droopy shorts that reached down to his knees. All he needed was a floppy mouser, dubbined boots and a bladder football. He could have been mistaken for the inside right of the Wanderers the year they won the FA cup.

His evening shower was a routine he stuck to rigidly. He was very keen on cleanliness. Not only his own, but that of others too. Robbie was not a great one for showering, it has to be said, at least when he was acutely unwell, and he soon developed a noticeable hum. Stand by him in the queue at the hatch and it didn't take you long to detect the faint aroma of performing seals. Simon sat by him one night at the TV, and after a moment or two his nostrils started to twitch. He turned and looked at Robbie, then addressed him in words none of the staff would have cared – or dared – to use.

'Robbie, man. It's time you had a bath. You're starting to smell like a kipper's fanny.'

Clyde and I smirked, then tensed ourselves, waiting for Robbie's onslaught. But he didn't lash out. He looked for a long time at Simon with that dead-eye glare of his, and then slowly a smile seeped across his face.

'You're a cheeky bastard,' he said.

Sometimes, in the ward mail, we would receive warnings about dangerous persons who might be in our vicinity – patients on the run from other parts of the UK, for example. We usually left them to Charlie to read and file, but I was bored in the office one time and flicked through the post. There was a circular from an NHS trust in Bristol, warning of the behaviour of a former patient of theirs, who was something of an itinerant barker, but a dangerous one. He had a thing about IPCUs, secure units and high-security hospitals. He liked to get himself in there and cause ructions. The circular gave his name, but also stated that he often used aliases, and sometimes called himself Tiger. He was One to Watch, they said. 'Mmmm, I thought, one man's One to Watch is another man's handful.' And I slid the circular into the folder of such things.

A month or so later, Luke and I returned from our evening meal in the canteen to find that the ward had gained an admission in our absence. The police had brought a man in after he 'went berresk', in Gordon's phrase, in the shopping centre. The admission was in the Smoke Room, sitting alone. He was tall and thin, wearing a black coat and a black beanie. His lantern jaw was gritty with black stubble. He did not look like the kind of man you'd be glad to see your lassie bring home.

'What do we know about him?' I aked John.

'Tony Stiles. Manc accent. Bad attitude.'

'Says it all,' said Gordon.

Dr Bankstreet was not available. So Charlie had bleeped the SHO to come and interview him, clerk him in. Now the patient stood up from his seat, flicked his fag end at the ashtray and headed out. Charlie joined us.

'Tony,' he said, 'the duty doc will be here as soon as he can.'

'Yeah, right. I just want to get some shut-eye. You got a bed round here?'

'Sure. You're in Room 2. Dennis will show you where it is.'

Stiles got his eye on me, nodded and headed off up the corridor.

'Stick with him,' Charlie whispered to me. 'Try and keep him up there.'

'Right.'

I caught up with him and edged slightly ahead.

'Room's this way, Tony,' I said.

He made no answer but when we came to the Nurses' Station sat down on a seat there and took a baccy tin from his pocket.

'Your room's this one,' I said.

'Just gonna have a smoke before I hit the sack.'

'You can't smoke up here.'

'There's an ashtray here.'

'Yeah. Shouldn't be. If you want to smoke, you have to do it in the Smoke Room.'

He looked directly at me. They say the eyes are the windows of the soul. This guy needed no spiritual Windolene.

'Listen, you bald-headed cunt. I want a smoke. And I don't intend to go all the way back down there for one.'

'So you can't have one then.' (I don't know where the courage for that came from.) 'Unless you want to go out into the courtyard.'

John arrived.

'Duty doc's here,' he said.

The SHO at the time was an Indian chap called Sunil. He was tall, handsome, cultured and one of the most agreeable people you could hope to meet. When John and I accompanied Stiles into the Interview Room, Sunil was seated in one of the chairs. He immediately stood up and with a broad smile offered Stiles his hand.

'Mr Stiles,' he said.

'Fuck off, Paki,' was Stiles's spat response.

'Oy, sir!' I snapped. Disgust at any form of racist insult is another of the many big bees in my empty big head. 'Have a little respect.'

'Or what?' snarled Stiles.

'Or else,' said John, stepping between us.

Stiles gave a superior scoff.

'Sorry, mate. Just don't like Pakis.'

'The doctor is Indian, not Pakistani,' I said.

'Same difference, mate.' Stiles shrugged.

Sunil dismissed this trivia with a shake of his head.

'Please, Mr Stiles, sit down,' he said.

Stiles did so with ill grace. Sunil sat down too, with his back to me. John sat by Stiles. I stood behind Sunil's chair so that Stiles was facing me directly. It wasn't a smart move. I have no recollection of what Sunil asked him, although I could hazard a guess. The format rarely changed. Nor do I remember what Stiles said. And the reason for that is quite simple. All the time Sunil spoke to him, Stiles was staring coldly at me. I held his eye at first, through some misguided macho desire not to let him think he had me cowed. But the more I held his eye, the more he stared. And the icier the glare became. It wasn't long before I knew in my innermost being that this man wanted to do me in. And not just kill me. Torture me. Suck the marrow from my bones. Do all sorts of weird shit to me before he let my soul escape. I was looking into the eyes of a psychopath, I told myself. And goading him by doing so.

And then I realised, all at once, who was sitting before me.

The session ended without any resolution. Sunil said he would let Dr Bankstreet decide in the morning. We left the interview room. Stiles turned for Room 2.

'Go up with him, Denny, will you?' said John. 'I've my dinner to get yet. I'll send Lukey up as well.'

Excellent. Alone in an empty corridor with a man who wanted my tripes for toad-in-the-hole. A stratagem was called for.

'Listen, Tony,' I said. 'I think you and I might have got off on the wrong foot about the smoking thing. It's just, you know, regs, man.'

'Yeah? Don't worry about it, mate,' he said. 'You can call me Tiger.'

When Luke came up, Tony the Tiger was already on his bed. I left Luke to keep guard and went down to the office. Charlie and Sunil were there, writing up notes.

'Sorry about that racist shite,' I said to Sunil.

'Think nothing of it.'

'I know who this joker is,' I said.

Charlie looked up. 'Yeah?'

'Yeah,' I said, taking down the folder and removing the circular in question. 'There's our man.'

Charlie studied the paper then passed it on to Sunil.

'We'll need to keep an eye on Mr Stiles,' Charlie said.

'Dr Bankstreet should be notified,' said Sunil.

'Yep. She'll probably discharge him in the morning.'

And so it was done. Next day Dr Bankstreet interviewed him with John and Luke present. The interview took ten minutes. Then Tony the Tiger was kicked out.

'Bad,' said Dr Bankstreet as she returned to the office. 'But not mad.'

Psychopaths are rarer in life than they are in fiction, and very different too. The profession doesn't like the term and doesn't use it any more, preferring the newer description 'antisocial personality disorder'. A psychopath by any other name would smell as dangerous. Characteristics of a psychopath include the inability to form or maintain personal relationships, difficulty in experiencing or showing emotions and a marked absence of empathy with others. They have difficulty with normal feelings of compassion, shame, remorse and guilt. Nothing is ever their fault. But they can often be charming and pleasant on the surface.

Psychopath or 'patient suffering from antisocial personality disorder' – I'd met one when I met Stiles. We were lucky he wasn't with us long enough to cause any ructions.

32

First be thou void of these affections,
Compassion, love, vain hope and heartless fear,
Be moved at nothing, see thou pity none,
But to thyself smile when the Christians moan.

Christopher Marlowe, *The Jew of Malta*

And then we got Lawrence. As if having Sniff, Elaine, Terry, Barry and Simon on the ward at the one time – with a wee flying visit from Tiger – were not enough, we got Lawrence. Lawrence was the final touch, the last lick of varnish, the cherry on the top. He was a Londoner but had moved up and lived in the city for some time. He had probably, however, come slowly northwards and only moved on from each location as the population found out about him. He was extremely mad and extremely violent. He came out to us as the culmination of a bizarre series of events.

He had taken ill again while working on a building site and seriously assaulted a gaffer, for which he was admitted to the psychie ward in the city hospital. While in there he was hurt in an accident and required surgery. During his operation the drapes (sterile coverings for protection during operations) around his neck caught fire and his neck was fairly badly burned. Something to do with swabbing alcohol catching fire after a cauterising tool had been switched on. When Lawrence woke up and discovered what had happened, he was a little put out. In fact, he was very put out. He went on the rampage and trashed the ward he was in, causing thousands of pounds' worth of damage. He was snared and brought out to Ward 25.

This was the most impressive arrival of any patient I ever saw in all my time on the ward. Forget the Queen of Sheba. Handel couldn't write a sinfonia impressive enough for this operatic appearance. There were six men on duty that day: Charlie, Clyde, John, Luke, Gordon and me, as well as four females: Pamela, Geraldine, Rona and Ursula. We were all fairly wrought up by the time Lawrence arrived, Charlie having heard something of his backstory from the Charge Nurse in the city hospital and having relayed it to us.

Two police motorcycle riders preceded the ambulance and a police car tailed it. When the two paramedics in the front seat of the ambulance got out and opened the back door, three male orderlies piled out. They slid out an easy-lift ambulance trolley. On it was the patient, strapped to it in several places and unconscious. An anaesthetist came out last. Lawrence hadn't just been sedated for his trip; he had been anaesthetised. They were taking no chances.

'Fuck me,' said John as we stood and watched this performance. 'Who is this guy? Hannibal Lecter?'

And if they had brought Lawrence out on a gurney, wearing a metal face mask and a straitjacket, as Lecter is in *The Silence of the Lambs*, it could not have made a bigger impression. This guy had to be a management problem. Sorry, a handful.

'Bit over the top?' Charlie said smilingly to the nurse in charge of the transfer.

'You think? Wait till this guy wakes up. You fellas are gonnae be busy.'

He was wheeled into Room 4, the one in the faraway corner, and transferred, still unconscious, into the bed. His escort left. Charlie assigned two men to special him. To be nursed in his room exclusively, meals to be taken in there too. He hadn't regained consciousness by the time we went home.

Next morning Lawrence was awake. We could hear him bawling as we entered the ward from the Buffer Zone. His London twang was bounding off the walls.

'GET ME SAHM PINEKILLAHS AWR OI'LL KILL YOU MAVVAHFACKAHS!'

I slipped off my jacket and went with John to Room 4, to relieve the night shift.

'LET ME AHT A THIS COFFIIIIN!'

'If I could get him into a fuckin' coffin,' growled Les from the night shift, 'he wouldn't be gettin' out in a hurry.'

'You're welcome to this, boys,' said the other bloke, and they left.

John stood in the doorway and gave Lawrence a frank stare. I stood behind John and looked round his shoulder. Lawrence was an overweight man with lank, greasy hair. He sat up in bed, propped against three pillows.

'WOT THE FACK A YOU LOOKIN' EHT?'

'Don't be like that, Lawrence,' said John. 'I could be really good for you.'

'FACK AWFF, YOU SCADDISH CANT!'

'Now, now, Lawrie,' said John. 'You'll hurt your throat if you shout like that.'

'FACK MY FROWT!'

'Tsk, tsk. Sounds like a London gay club.'

'GET ME SAHM PINEKILLAHS! OYM IN EGGONEE!'

'Well,' said John, 'if you pipe down a little, and stop being so aggressive, I'll see what we can do.'

'FACK YEW, MITE, YOR AVIN A LAWRFF!'

'Up to you, Loz,' said John, sitting down in the armchair at the door. 'A little courtesy goes a long way.'

'YOR AVIN A LAWRFF!'

The dialogue got a little repetitive at this point, and stayed that way until Luke and Gordon came up to take a spell and allow us to receive the night report from Charlie.

'Universal precautions,' muttered Luke as we left. 'He's fizzin'.'

I soon found out what that meant. Lawrence had woken up in the small hours and had been as obstreperous with the night shift as he was now being with us: shouting, threatening, demanding. At one point he had attempted to force his way out of the room and had been restrained by four men and jagged, then returned to his bed. The dope hadn't touched him.

However, apart from any physical threat that he represented, he was also effervescent with HIV, Hep C and various other unpleasant letter combinations. Nor was he averse to spitting, oh no. Not Lawro; he liked a hawk, a hiss and a slobber. I don't know if anyone has ever spat at you – I sincerely hope not – but it's one of the most unpleasant things that can happen to you. It's not just a little *tph* of white saliva, usually. The assailant generally drags up a clot of knuckly phlegm from as far down as he can, and gobs it at you like an Amerindian native with a poison dart. With somebody as full of diseases as Lawrence, it would be six and half a dozen which was the more toxic. Personally, I think I'd take my chances with the poison dart.

So we had to take what are called 'universal precautions'. These are basically common-sense ways of dressing to avoid contamination or infection. Anyone coming into contact of any kind with Lawrence had to wear a barrier gown of lightweight polypropylene that tied at the back of the neck and the waist, and had elasticated cuffs. Latex gloves and a spit guard completed the kit. The spit guard was a face shield that consisted of a sheet of a thin plastic film called Mylar, held in place by an elastic band round the head, and a foam forehead cushion. Togged up in all this plastic and latex finery, a nurse had the look of a mad scientist or maybe a singularly hygienic knight. But the precautions were absolutely necessary. Lawrence thought nothing of dragging a green and yellow grogger up from the soles of his feet and flubbering it at whoever was in range. The Mylar shields were often dribbling with his infected slaver. It was a form of germ warfare. We all loved him dearly.

Once a day the guys would escort him out of the room and seat him in an armchair at the door while another nurse, usually another guy, went in and changed the bedlinen and towels. Then he was escorted back into the room. Meals were taken under the same guard. One nurse brought the tray and set it on the table then left, before the nurses on obs allowed Lawrence out of the bed and anywhere near it.

But there were problems. Using so many staff on one patient was bad for the ward. There was a proportionate shortage of attention on other people. And other people weren't the most sedentary or biddable of bodies themselves. Robbie. Simon. The usual suspects. So Charlie had to have recourse to agency staff to beef up the numbers. And agency staff, like a Number 11 batsman, are a bit hit and miss. Some are superb. Some are, frankly, duff.

It was one such duffer who got himself badly hurt one morning. Luke and I had been specialing Lawrence until breakfast.

'OIM SHORE OI DOWNT NOW WOT YOU FINK YOU LOOK LIKE IN VEM FACKIN TOGS, MITE! YOR AVIN A LAWRFF!'

Then two agency nurses, one a dunderheid with a ponytail and a hide full of tattoos, and the other with a face full of metal, came to spell us.

'Fucksake,' said Luke as we headed out of the ward and up to the canteen, 'Painted Boy and Piercings Boy. How did they ever get on an agency list?'

'Maybe they're good enough nurses,' I said. I could be quite positive when out of the ward and heading for a bacon roll.

They weren't. When we got back we found Lawrence out of the door of his room and swinging a metal stand at them. This was for the orange bags used in hospitals for waste disposal. It consisted of a metal base, upright and lip round which the fabric of the bag was wrapped, under a metal lid. It wasn't too hefty but it was awkward and full of sharp angles. Lawrence had grabbed hold of the one outside his room, where we disposed of anything he had soiled, and was now wielding it against these two numpties.

'CAM AHEAD, YOU FACKIN NENCIES! OI'LL CLEAVE YER OWPEN!'

The two nurses were stepping back as he swung the stand at them in a wide semicircle, then stepping forward to try to reason with him.

'Get in tight to him!' yelled Luke. 'Don't let him swing it!'

'Eh?' said the dipshit with the tattoos.

'Don't let him swing it!'

Painted Boy stepped forward just as Lawrence swung the stand again, and took it square in the pan. His cheek split like a dry log. I set my alarm off. Then Luke and I waited until Lawrence was at the extremity of the semicircle and went in under the sweep, flattening him against the wall.

'CANTS!'

When John came running with Clyde, Luke and I had Lawrence in the position and Johnny Staple Face was on his legs. At last someone else got to be bum man. Lawrence was none too graciously returned to his bed and spiked. The guy with tattoos was walked up to A & E to get the old herringbone stitch.

Charlie talked to Dr Bankstreet that afternoon. He said the presence of Lawrence on the ward was causing all sorts of logistical problems and that the care offered to other patients was suffering as a result of his male staff's concentration on nursing – actually guarding – Lawrence. The doc agreed she would speak to the people at the Big Hoose. One of their consultants came up and, dressed in the barrier stuff, interviewed Lawrence. He was moved the following weekend.

So the State Hospital got two of ours in the space of a week or two. We still had Robbie and Barry. And Simon, who was maintaining his equilibrium pretty well at the time. But I was getting tired, dog tired, of all the hassle. Tired as shit. Old-timer, plumb tuckered out.

I said to Charlie, 'I thought you didn't need me to help with the fighting.'

'Ah, this isn't fighting.'

'It sure as fuck isnae The Minister's Cat, anyway,' I said and headed off for a gasp.

I left Charlie staring at me in a puzzled manner.

In the Smoke Room John suddenly said, 'I know who that tattooed fucker is! Luke, you mind that guy, what was his name . . . Roddy somethin'?'

'Roddy the Body?'

'Aye, mind. He's tattooed all over his body. He used to work up in the adolescent ward, years ago.'

'Och aye,' said Luke. 'Polish surname?'

'Him,' agreed John. 'That's who the fucker is! He didnae have long hair at the time. Mind, he showed us. Everythin' up tae his neck, his wrists an' his ankles is tattooed.'

'Aye. The Technicolor nurse.'

'Told us his girl was the same. Tattoos everywhere. Tits and all.'

'Imagine them at it, eh? Like watchin' two rolls a wallpaper shaggin'.'

That lightened me a little before I went home. But only for the briefest of times.

33

The cross that some people have to bear through life is more onerous than we can ever know, the agony of it deriving from the fact that often it was thrust onto their shoulders in childhood by someone they loved and trusted. Someone who should have been protecting them in their vulnerability. Someone who should have been safeguarding their every step through the one part of their lives that might reasonably be expected to be free from care, grief and pain. Hell knows, there's enough of that waiting for us in adulthood.

One of the bleakest and most dispiriting things about work on the Locked Ward was the regularity with which we had to nurse victims of CSA – child sexual abuse. A staggering number of women and also one or two men over the course of my seven and a half years on the ward were there because they could not cope with the crushing emotions that were left them as a hideous residue of their exploitation as children. Their abusers might be anyone – neighbours, babysitters, friends – but more probably, statistically, members of their own family: uncles, cousins, brothers or fathers. In one case at least, a mother. Recent high-profile cases in the media have shown that females abuse children sexually too. It is far less common than among males, but real enough nonetheless. We knew that from the experience of nursing the victims.

Adults who have been sexually abused as children may suffer from anxiety, depression, low self-esteem and post-traumatic stress disorder. This latter, most commonly associated in the public mind with soldiers and the after-effects of war, is a serious anxiety disorder that can arise after any traumatic event. This might be the horrors of war, certainly; but it might equally be the horror of childhood sexual abuse. The victim may relive the original events in nightmares or through flashbacks. Further complications can include problems with adult relationships, promiscuity, alcohol and/or substance abuse, self-harm, crime and suicide.

The likelihood, the extreme likelihood, is that the closer the relationship with the abuser, the more severely harmed will be the victim. Sexual abuse by a member of the family, as in father/daughter incest, results in serious long-term psychological damage. However, it is not more likely, as is sometimes thought, to result in the victim abusing his or her own children. Most adult victims of CSA do not go on to be offenders themselves. Few adult offenders report sexual abuse in their own childhood. So no causal link can be assumed.

The treatment for a CSA victim normally depends on the problem presenting itself at the time. For example, a victim suffering from depression would be treated for that, although familiarity with the case history would always be taken into account. Sometimes Cognitive Restructuring techniques would be used to address the deeper-seated issue. (These are therapies for understanding what causes negative or stressful emotions, and then addressing them in a way that will allow the victim to come to terms with them and, ultimately, turn them round.)

One thing I must mention here that I thought decidedly strange. During my time in Care of the Elderly I nursed an old man who was severely demented. His notes recorded that he had regularly sexually abused his daughters – and sons – throughout their childhood. Unconditional nursing. I nursed him as I did any other man on the ward. Not only did his daughters visit him regularly, but they brought their own children, some of them only toddlers, to visit him too. It was not common for little children to be on that ward. Whether his sons ever visited, I cannot honestly say; I remember none. But I wondered how women who had been abused as children could bring their own kids into the company of their abuser.

Over the course of my time on the Locked Ward, I came to know many female victims. Some required to be specialed, some did not. One was abused by a stepfather, another by the friend of her older brother and at least one, sadly, by her father.

'If a wee lassie cannae trust her father, what man can she bloody trust?'

'Yeh. Fathers should remember that. A daughter is gonnae judge every man she meets by her father. That's the template she's going to use, whether she knows it or not.'

'At least till she's old enough to differentiate.'

'I just don't have that gene. Thank God.'

'Most of us don't.'

'Yeah, I mean the gene even to begin to understand that behaviour.'

It wasn't a topic that encouraged much chit-chat among us staff, but that exchange took place over a meal before we moved on to other topics. Our female colleagues, especially Pamela and Geraldine, the trained nurses, did a lot of work with these women. Over a long period of time they built up a relationship with them. At first it would be a purely professional one, albeit with a very human and sympathetic face. Gradually, a degree of trust would form. Pam or Geraldine might then suggest a series of one-to-one interviews for disclosure. Slowly, hesitantly, maybe even reluctantly, patients would start to discuss their thoughts, their feelings and their problems, including the one that was responsible for their being there. After some time they might tentatively broach the underlying topic of the abuse. I believe that progress was always uncertain and slow. Nonetheless, progress there undoubtedly was, in some cases.

There were many, however, where there was hardly any progress worthy of the name. Some patients were discharged from time to time and attempted to forge a life in the outside world, only to be readmitted regularly. Some were inpatients for years. Other treatments were tried with specific patients. Eye Movement Desensitisation and Reprocessing (EMDR) was one such process I saw used. Emotional Freedom Therapy (EFT) another, although some sneer at this as being pseudoscientific hokum.

EMDR basically consists of the victim focusing on an object moving from side to side while concentrating on an image representing the trauma. This should take place somewhere quiet that represents safety to the patient, and (s)he should have in mind an image or memory that represents happiness or security, which (s)he can go to quickly, in time of need. The rapid movement of the eyes is thought to bring about changes in the brain that may help desensitise a traumatic memory by helping the patient to recall it without being disturbed by it, and then reprocess it into acceptance. Or, as it's been neatly summarised: 'I can't deal with it' becomes 'It happened. I'll get over it.'

I've been present at several sessions of EMDR and can attest that sometimes it can have a very positive outcome. Once, however, with a male patient, the process obviously shone too bright a light into a dark place too quickly, and he became extremely distressed. He screamed, stood up and kicked chairs over, then burst into uncontrollable sobs. We had to terminate the session at once and get him to concentrate on his safe place. We walked him quickly to his room, and after half an hour he was calmer. To his eternal credit, once he explained that he had got a flash of what had happened, a flash that was burning in its intensity, far too intense for him to be able to deal with at that point, he said he would like to go on with the therapy another day. This is what I admired most about so many of the patients: their sheer, resolute courage. Daily they fought demons, dragons and all sorts of horrors, and yet, after every defeat, minor or significant, they squared their shoulders and faced up to the adversary again.

EFT consists of tapping acupuncture points (meridians) on the head and face while focusing on the trauma. I've sat and watched patients tap rhythmically with the tips of their fingers on the forehead, eyebrows, bridge of the nose, upper lip and chin, cheekbones, temples and so on. While they were doing this, they were to think about the trauma. The theory was that it would gradually lose its power to terrify; they would come to terms with it and move on. Some think that any benefit of the therapy is simply due to the positive aspect of having someone kind and concerned listen and care. I did see some people benefit from it, but I always thought of it as 'Pat-a-cake, pat-a-cake'. I suppose I'm just naturally sceptical.

I tried writing therapy with some victims of CSA, again with mixed success. Some found it impossible even to attempt; others took to it like a duck to oranges. One woman, who had lost all access to her children over the years, the result of a sorry succession of substance misuse, alcoholism and prostitution, asked if she could write the story of her life from adolescence. But nobody had to read it. She only wanted the exercise of writing it. I agreed, of course. Perhaps the writing would prove cathartic enough in itself. I used to sit in the GP Room doing the crossword while she typed on the PC and saved her writing to her own disk. Another, younger, woman wrote poems and short prose pieces that touched distantly upon her trauma. Again I told her no one need see her work, but she showed me some poems. Some of her imagery was startling. However, she stopped abruptly after a few weeks, saying that it was bringing it all back to her and she couldn't cope. It was a great pity. She had the poetic eye.

I took her out for a walk one autumn morning, early, when mist was just clearing from the ground. Every shrub and hedge was draped with spider's webs, beaded with droplets of water, glistening in the leaves. She nudged me. 'Look.' She smiled, pointing at the webs. 'The fairies have spread their washing out to dry.' I know. The image is sugary enough to induce Type 2 Diabetes by itself. But it's clever. Hardly surprising; the girl was as sharp as a semitone above pitch. CSA isn't confined to stupid people. No mental illness is.

Not all cases were resistant to therapy, however. One woman, perhaps the least likely to succeed in many eyes, managed to deal with her problems and was discharged to a tenancy in a local village. There she met a man and started to go out with him. Within the year they were married. And still are. She hasn't required medication in all that time.

And the generosity of spirit of people lost in the darkest, most impenetrable jungles of their own minds never failed to amaze me. One young woman, a CSA victim, required close obs at all times. Usually patients in these circumstances prefer to be specialed by a female nurse, for obvious reasons. This girl didn't, and I often spent an hour in a chair by her door, keeping an eye open for attempts at self-harm. We built up a bond, to the extent that she told me some of her story. Not all by any means, but still some details that appalled me. Often I was at a loss to know how to react, what to say, how to try to help her come to terms with those things. I was open with her, though, and told her that I wished I could do more to help her. As a man, I would have liked to have been able to say something that helped her in some small way, however negligible, to deal with the intolerable burden another man had placed on her.

One night, as I was sitting listening to her, Rona came round the corner and told me I had an urgent phone call. It was my brother. My father had died. I told Geraldine and she instructed me to go home straight away. I went back and explained the situation to Rona, who had taken over on obs from me. Rona gave me a hug and said she was sorry.

'I'm really sorry to hear that too, Dennis,' said the girl in the room. 'You must go home and be with your family. They need you more than we do now. I'll say a prayer for you. And listen. Thanks; you *do* make a difference.'

34

Such is the course salt sallow lust doth run.
John Marston, *The Malcontent*

It could be difficult for these women when certain types of male patients were on the ward – the kind of men whose illnesses manifested themselves in sexual disinhibition or even sexual aggression. I don't mean men like Edward, whose nature was frankly sexual and who enjoyed sex openly whenever he could. Some of his behaviour might have been inappropriate in the circumstances he found himself in, but he was not what one female patient called a 'sleazeball'. He did not talk inappropriately to females, make inappropriate overtures or strike women as a threat. Some others, unfortunately, did.

Barry was one such. Whether it was true or not that he had arrived on the ward to hide from justice, he had kept a relatively low profile at first but began to show his horns. Maybe he was feeling more secure from capture. In any case, he was soon fractious with staff and with Dr Bankstreet. He carped and complained about the slightest thing: meds not doled out on time, nobody going to the filling station when it suited his convenience, even that the wrong meals were being delivered to him. It made no difference when we pointed out that *he* ordered his meals, or when we showed him the detached section that accompanied every meal, torn from the menu he had completed himself the day before. He accused staff of rewriting his order. He said people were going into his room and stealing things, notably his fags. He accused certain staff of favouritism, mumping that nobody ever had any time for him. Whether he had genuinely been ill on admission, it was certain he was getting ill now. He became violent towards another patient one evening and was restrained and injected by the night shift. The following morning just after we had arrived on shift, he lurched out of his room naked and fell sideways against a wall.

'Barry!' roared Rona. 'Get back in there and get dressed!'

'YOUSE'VE FUCKED MAH HEAD UP! MAH HEAD'S FULL A COTTON WOOL!' he yelled.

'Get in and get dressed!'

He grabbed his genitals and wagged them lewdly in Rona's direction. 'You, ya fuckin' bitch! You'd love it!'

John and Luke sprinted up and grabbed him by an arm each.

'That's enough a that! Any more and you'll get your arse jagged for you.'

'Fuckin' jags! Mah head's full a cotton wool!'

They huckled him back into his room. Half an hour later, as we were serving breakfast, and the domestics were going about their mopping and hoovering business, he re-emerged from his room like a bear with a sore arse and stomped along the corridor to the Dining Area. At least he was fully dressed this time.

'WHERE'S MAH BREAKFAST?' he bellowed at the hatch.

Gordon looked out. 'Just a minute, Barry. Didn't know you were there.'

'SEE WHAT AH FUCKIN' MEAN? ALL FOR EVERYBODY ELSE. WELL YOUSE CAN ALL FUCK OFF!'

He about-turned and barged into one of the wee domestic ladies practising a few artistic passes with a Hoover.

'SAME GOES FOR YOU, BITCH!'

He jabbed both hands against her shoulders and thrust her against a wall. The back of her head smacked against it with a sickening thud and she screamed. Barry took off for his room, but Clyde, John and Luke were equal to the chase. Clyde decked him with a flying tackle and then all three dragged him to his feet and hauled him off to the Treatment Room. Their progress was so precipitate that Barry came into contact with a door frame on the way. Nobody apologised. Charlie shouted for me and Gordon. So all six males were in the Treatment Room with Barry. Charlie started to draw a jag up.

'What's this you're givin' me?'

'Acuphase,' replied Charlie. 'You're written up for it. You need it. You're getting it.'

'Ah don't want that,' spat Barry. 'Let's see what else you've got. ' He craned his neck to look in the drugs trolley.

'It's no a shop, pal,' said Charlie and shut the lid. Then he stood before Barry with his dish full of needles. 'Now, you know why I'm giving you this?'

'Nawt.'

'I'm giving you this because you are becoming increasingly hostile and aggressive. I won't stand for staff being assaulted on this ward. Especially non-nursing staff. That wee lady has nothing to do with your care and was just going about her job of making this place more comfortable for you. You were inappropriate with Rona this morning. You shouted at Gordon at breakfast. You assaulted wee Bella. Three strikes and you're out. Now, are you going to take this without being restrained?'

'AHM AH FUCK!'

'Boys?' said Charlie.

John, Luke and Clyde grabbed him, marched him over to the couch in the corner, and stood him facing it. Clyde and John braced their legs against the backs of his calves so that he could not easily kick back. I reached round, unbuckled his belt and pulled his jeans down. He farted.

'That woulda put a nice partin' in your hair, if you'd had any,' said Luke.

'Dirty bastard!'

'I don't think a fart is an offensive weapon,' Charlie said grimly. 'Right.'

'I don't know,' I said, standing back.

The guys inclined his upper half forward and Charlie stepped forward and lanced him.

'Now,' said Charlie, stepping back, 'the guys are going to walk you to your room. You stay there for a while until you calm down. Dennis?'

I readjusted Barry's clothing and the Three Musketeers walked him back to his room. He put up a token struggle, flexing his arms, cursing and so on, but no more than that. They laid him on his bed and shut the door behind them. Muffled blessings could be heard as they walked away.

'Keep an eye on that door for half an hour,' said Charlie. 'After that, he'll be in dreamland.'

And so it turned out. Acuphase is a hefty dunt in anybody's taxonomy of hits. Barry slept round a complete clock. He got up the next day in the mid-morning, silent and surly, still woozy from the dope in his body. I offered to make him a coffee and a sandwich. He nodded agreement and ate his meal quietly in the Dining Area alone. After that, he made his way to the Smoke Room. Ten minutes later, as I sat in the office with Luke and Charlie, a girl called Yvonne came to the door and knocked.

'Yvonne,' said Charlie, 'what can we do for you?'

'It's Barry,' she said. 'He's talking filth in the Smoke Room to the lassies.'

'Is he now?'

'He told me I needed a shag. Said he would like to give me a good seeing-to.'

Luke and I stood up and crossed the corridor to the Smoke Room. Barry was sitting hunched forward, his elbows on his knees, a fag stuck between two fingers of his right hand.

'What you been sayin' to these women?' I asked him.

'Nuthin'.'

'He said he needed a ride,' said a girl by the window.

'And he told me he'd give me a good time,' added Yvonne from behind Luke.

'He's a dirty bastard,' said an older woman opposite him. 'He wouldnae say these things if you boys were around.'

'All I says, right,' protested Barry, 'was that I hadnae had my hole in months. It's awright for you cunts. Gettin' plenty. Gettin' it regular. It's nuthin' wrong. It's only natural. Everybody does it.'

'It might be natural,' I said, 'but talking filth to these women isn't. They're entitled to come in here and have a smoke without being upset or pestered by folk like you.'

'What the fuck are you?' sneered Barry. 'Germaine fuckin' Greer?'

'I'm impressed,' I replied. 'You should read her book. Maybe teach you a few things. Just cut the dirty crack when women are around.'

'Fuck you, baldy. They're only fuckin' bitches. They love it. It gets them goin'. In the mood—'

'Right! Out,' said Luke.

'What?'

'Nip your fag and fuck off out of here.'

'You serious?'

'Serious all right. Get weavin'. And don't come back in here today if there's women in.'

'Fuckin' hell!'

Barry nipped his smoke, dropped the red tip in the ashtray and slouched out, muttering under his breath. Luke and I closed the door and stood watching him go up the corridor. He turned right, into the Dayroom. I let out an exasperated sigh. Luke agreed.

And then Rona screamed from the Dayroom. Her scream was closely followed by the alarm sounding and a girl called Betty running from the Dayroom and down the corridor, crying. We took off. Charlie looked out of the office. John came sprinting down from the bedded area.

'He's gropin' Rona!' wept Betty.

Luke and I got there just before Charlie but just after John. Rona was scarlet, spitting with rage and weeping at the insult. She was also trying to gouge Barry's eyes out with her nails. John got him by the shoulder and wrenched him away from her. Luke and Charlie grabbed him.

'Pam! Take Rona and make her a cup a tea!' Charlie said. I'd never noticed Pamela arriving.

I followed the others as they herded Barry back through to his room. They flung him on the bed.

'Keep him here,' hissed Charlie and went away to draw something up.

'Oh, you've fucked up good this time,' whispered John into his ear.

'She was askin' for it!' snapped Barry.

'That's a colleague and a friend of ours,' said John.

'A married woman and a mother,' said Luke. 'Your whole attitude to women stinks.'

Charlie came back with another dunt. Barry offered no resistance. I went down to the GP Room, where Pamela was sitting with Rona. Rona had her palms round a large mug of tea. She had composed herself.

'How are you, hen?' I asked.

'I'm all right, Dennis,' said Rona. 'That dirty get. I hope Charlie jagged him.'

'With a blunt needle full of Paraquat, I think,' I said. She laughed a little. 'What did he do?'

'Oh, he came into the Dayroom as I was going out. Stuck his tongue out and waggled it at me. Told me what he was going to do with it. I told him to dream on. Then he grabbed me, licked my face and stuck his hand between my legs.'

'Dirty get,' I agreed.

'Poor wee Betty,' said Rona. 'She got a hell of a fright, wee sowel. She was awfu' upset.'

'She was,' I agreed.

'Betty'll be all right,' Pamela said. 'As long as you are, hen, that's the main thing.'

'Ach, I'm fine. I just got a fright, that's all. It's nae mair than Ian does on a Friday night after a skinful.' She laughed.

Barry was put on close any time he emerged from his room. He drew his horns in a little. He was still unpleasant and morose but offered no more direct affronts to women. He was creepy though; there was no doubt. He also had a stash of eye-wateringly hard-core porn. It only came to light when we carried out a room-to-room search for illegal drugs.

'Come and take a look at this,' said John.

'Fuckin' hell! Where did he get this?' I said. We called Charlie.

'How did he get a hold of this?' asked Charlie.

'Visitor probably.'

'Visitor? The only visitor he gets is his mother. You think she brings this shit in under the Jaffa Cakes?'

'Nobody else visits him,' I said.

'No, but other patients have visitors. Other patients go out. Somebody has brought him this stuff. And it isn't his mother.'

'He's bad enough without all this,' observed John.

'Right,' said Charlie. 'This stuff's impounded. Clear it out and lock it in the Dookits for the time being.'

Barry was not chuffed when he found out.

'You can't just confiscate my magazines.'

'Oh yes I can,' Charlie answered. 'There are women on this ward, staff as well as patients. You have a bad enough attitude. It's not at all appropriate that you should have this material while you're in here.'

'Well, I want it returned when I go.'

Charlie looked at him. 'All right. If it's still here when you go.'

Barry didn't like it one little bit, but there was nothing he could do.

Clive, an inpatient many years before my spell on the ward, was brought back in from the city hospital, unwell. Among many other things, he was accused of propositioning two schoolgirls on the top deck of a bus and then exposing himself to them when they contemptuously rejected his advances. He agreed that he was guilty of talking to them and suggesting sex, but not of flashing. After a fight in the hospital he was brought to us, but he wasn't with us a day before two uniformed officers from the city police came to investigate a charge made against him by a female patient. I sat in on the interview. The female officer conducted the questioning. She said that the patient accused him of sitting next to her in the Television Lounge and exposing himself.

'Nah,' said Clive. 'Didnae happen.'

'You didn't remove your penis from your trousers?'

'Nah. Didnae happen.'

'And you didn't begin to masturbate until stopped by a nursing assistant?'

'Nah. Didnae happen.'

'What *did* happen?'

'Aw, ah just had itchy ba's, ye know, so ah scratched them. That's it. Ah wisnae wankin', like. I'm sure you can tell the difference between scratchin' an' wankin', eh, officer?'

'So why would this woman accuse you of it?'

'Cos she's fuckin' mad, int she? She's in a loony bin.'

'The nursing assistant, Mr Thomson, says your penis was exposed.'

'Nah. Didnae happen. He's mistaken, int he?'

This was not untypical of Clive. There was a marked element of sleaze in his conversations with women. He liked to talk about sex, in detail, to them. Our colleagues would interrupt him sharply if he started any of that old snash with them. John had an especial animus against him; there was some previous from earlier admissions. But it wasn't only females that Clive liked to talk dirty with. There was a gay patient on the ward, a likeable little man called Frederick, who was bipolar. Well on the way to recovery by this time, Frederick would stroll up the ward to the Smoke Room, passing the time of day pleasantly with everyone he met. One or two of the more butch among the patient cohort jarred him about his sexuality in the early days.

'You a poof?'

'Well, like they say, it doesn't make you a bad person.'

'But are you a poof?'

'I don't like that word. It's ugly. It's an insult.'

'Well what word dae ye want us tae use? Bender? Bent shot? Homo?'

'No, no. None of these. Let's just say I'm a friend of Dorothy.'

'Dorothy whae?'

At the hatch his banter was always the same.

'Hello and good afternoon to you, young Dennis . . .' (Or Luke or John or Rona, whoever.) 'I'll treat myself to a cup of weak tea with a little milk, please. But no sugar.' Pause. 'Because I'm sweet enough as it is. Oh, and I'll be a devil and take a suggestive digestive.'

Everybody liked Frederick, even the hairy-knuckle brigade. Clive stood behind him at the hatch one day and watched his little routine. When Frederick turned away with his cuppa and suggestive biscuit, Clive spoke.

'Ah know what you're intae. Ah've never tried it masel, but ah bet you'd love tae get your hands on this dinky wee arse.'

'Don't flatter yourself,' Frederick retorted and flounced away. Frederick had a good flounce, a better flounce than tasselled silk curtains.

'Wait a wee minute, petal,' Clive called after him. 'Ah'll sit on your knee an' we'll see what comes up.'

'Shut it, you,' John growled in his ear. 'That's a decent wee man. Leave him alone.'

More serious was Jack. He was transferred to the IPCU from the acute ward upstairs because he had sexually assaulted a female patient. The girls sedulously avoided him. He didn't stay long with us. One morning we came in to start the diurnal grind at 7.30 and found him gone. He had attempted to rape one of the female patients, and although he hadn't succeeded, he had beaten her up rather badly. He was even then up in the Big Hoose – hopefully, as Luke said, experiencing the appropriate joy of a warder giving him a body-cavity search.

35

What mad pursuit? What struggle to escape?
John Keats, 'Ode on a Grecian Urn'

It wasn't often that a patient managed to escape from the
ward, but it did happen from time to time. Usually, the
airlock design of the Buffer Zone made this impossible.
The glass in the windows of the Dayroom and those
bedrooms that gave on to the grounds was unbreakable.
The only rooms with sliding windows were those which
looked on to the courtyard, and there was no point anyone
escaping into the courtyard because its walls were three
storeys high, consisted of the windows of many other
wards and were pretty much unscalable. Anybody trying
it would attract the interest of half the hospital as a rival to
Spiderman. The only door in the courtyard was the one
that took you back into the Locked Ward. Crazy golf for
humans. A breakout would have to be done in a different
way. Dan managed it.

The ward was boiling like a nest of ants one night. The
staff had had to deal with crisis after crisis. We had just
restrained one patient, jagged him and put him into his room
to meditate on the futility of seeking material happiness,
when a rammie broke out in the Dayroom. Two patients
were fighting. They were really going at it too: swapping
meaty blows and spilling plenty of house red. When Luke,
John and Clyde waded in to separate them, a third got

involved from outside the ring, and Gordon and I had to wrestle him off the maul. And wrestle is the operative word. We rolled about the floor with this man, who was heavy and sweaty and panting with the exertion, and then, making a supreme effort to throw us off, he shit himself.

'Woah!' Gordon gagged.

'Code Brown! Code Brown!'

We threw ourselves off him and Gordon set off his alarm. Charlie and Geraldine came lickety-split from the office. Eventually, among us all, we got the heavyweight boxers separated and sent to opposite corners of the ward, the other guy's boxers cleaned up, and meds handed out to all three. That's when the phone rang. It was Judy from Ward 42 upstairs. They had a male patient going off it up there and needed male backup.

Charlie had a quandary. There was no question of not sending support. That was one of the things we did: provide bodies to other wards in emergencies. The very real problem was that here, on 25, we had one patient already restrained and jagged for loud and continual verbal aggression, two guys who hated the sight of each other and were itching for a return bout, and another who resented the fact that Gordon and I had 'made' him soil his St Michael's. Any or all of them might kick off again at any moment. We needed muscle on the floor here too. In the end, Charlie dispatched me and Luke. John and Clyde were at opposite ends of the ward, keeping a weather eye on Ali and Frazier, while Gordon had a roving brief around the ward. Charlie had said to him, 'Gordon, look with care about the ward, and silence those whom this vile brawl distracted.' At least, it seems to me that was the gist of what he said. I may not have it verbatim.

So, Luke and I made our way, by corridor and lift, up to Ward 42, two flights above. When we arrived at the foyer, it seemed that all of the staff were around the Nurses' Station. One or two patients were there too. Judy approached us and mentioned the patient's name. Jock was someone I'd known in the pubs of my local village. He was a big man (weren't they all?) but had been something of a gentle giant when I'd known him. Now he had given up the Falling-Down Water and was a devotee of the Fragrant Weed. It hadn't been an improvement, considering what it had done to his mind. In the course of that afternoon he had become hostile and withdrawn to the extent that the ward's consultant, one Dr Marjorie Bankstreet, had ordered his removal to the IPCU. When informed of his new status, he had gone apeshit and refused to be nominated for membership of that exclusive club. The staff tried to wheedle him but had no wheedling spoons. He lost the plot and started to throw the furniture around. That was when Judy phoned Charlie. Most of 42's staff were female. Their one male was as much use as a chocolate teapot.

Now Jock was barricaded in their games-room-cum-lounge. Judy knocked. Jock's voice roared at her to go away. Judy opened the door and stuck her head in.

'It's just me, Jock.'

She retracted her head fairly smartly as a blue snooker ball whistled through the aperture and embedded itself in the opposite wall. Had she not ducked, it would have burned a smoking O-shaped hole through her head worth five points. Luke strode forward. I followed.

'Here, sir!' shouted Luke. Then he ducked as a red, a fizzing split-fingered fastball, whistled past his ear. 'Enough a that!'

Jock fished another ball – the yellow, I think – from the capacious pocket of the Barbour jacket he was wearing. He was about to show us his change-up. Luke made a breenge. Jock stepped one pace to the side and lifted a wooden chair which he looped over his arm and began swinging around his head.

'Come and get it,' he hissed.

Luke immediately armed himself with another, the only sensible course of action in the circumstances. It's the same thinking as the nuclear deterrent, really. Jock rattled the snooker balls in his pocket. I stepped out from behind Luke.

'Jock,' I said, 'what's all the rammie about?'

'Fuck off. Ah'm gaun tae nae Locked Ward.' Then he did a double take. 'That you, Dennis?'

'Aye, it's me, Jock.'

'What you daein' here?'

'I work in the Locked Ward.'

'You dae? Ah thought you were—'

'I was. But I stopped it. And now I work in the Locked Ward.'

'Fuckin' hell.'

'You may well be right.'

The long and the short of it was is that Jock calmed down, divested himself of his chair and magazine of snooker balls, and agreed to be escorted to Ward 25 so long as it was for one night only and so long as *I* escorted him. Sometimes it's useful being a man who takes a drink.

When we got back down to 25, there was something of a flap on, so much so that Jock's arrival was treated as fairly low key. He was greeted and shown his room by Pamela. Charlie came to Luke and me the minute we were through the airlock.

'Either of you seen Dan? He's nowhere to be seen.'

'No. He didn't come with us.'

'How d'you mean?' asked Luke. 'He's nowhere to be seen?'

'Just that. We've scoured the place high and low for him. He isn't on the ward. He must have got out.'

'How?'

'That's what I'd like to know. He isn't fuckin' Houdini; he must have got out the door. I thought maybe when you guys went upstairs . . .'

'Naw,' said Luke definitely. 'Nobody got out with us.'

Charlie shook his head and ordered another search of the ward. He was right: Dan was nowhere to be seen. Not in his room, not in anyone else's room, not in the Dayroom, the GP Room or the Smoke Room. Not in the Pool Room, the Treatment Room, the Laundry Room, the Dookits or any of the cupboards. Not in the office or the Charge Nurse's office, nor in any nook, cranny or corner of the courtyard. It was as if he'd drawn a huge circle on the wall with black paint, stepped into it and pulled the circle after him as he stepped through to the outside world.

'Has to have got out the door,' muttered Charlie. 'But how?'

'Anybody's keys or swipe missing?' suggested John.

We all checked. Gordon's keys were not to be found. Panic stations. Now we turned the ward upside down looking for those. Nowhere.

'When did you use them last?' asked Geraldine.

'Erm, when I opened the GP Room door for Stewart. Mind? When all that carry-on was goin' on.'

'Did you leave them in the door?' asked Charlie.

'Must have,' Gordon said shamefacedly.

'Pillock,' said Charlie and went straight to the office and the phone.

'It's okay, Gordon,' said Pamela. 'Could have happened to any of us, with all the fighting and things.'

Charlie knew what he was doing. Dan was not the most imaginative of men. Charlie phoned Dan's mother, who lived five minutes away. And, sure enough, he was there, toasting his sweaty socks in front of the fire and enjoying a plateful of Mum's roasted cheese.

'That's fine,' said Charlie. 'Some of the guys will come for him in ten minutes.'

Dan had come upon Gordon's abandoned keys, snagged them and, while the donnybrook was going on, had used them to slip out of the door and away. He'd told his mother that he was on a pass from the ward. John and Luke drove round and picked him up. Gordon got his keys back and a brows-down from Charlie.

'It's imperative that you know where your keys and swipes are at all times. This worked out okay. If it had been anybody else, they'd have been halfway to Manchester by now, and your keys in the burn. We'd a had to get Security to change the locks and the swipe. You would have been in deep doo-doo. Right up to your neck.'

'Sorry, Charlie, it was all the rammie—'

'I know what it was. And I understand that. But let it be a lesson. Always guard keys and swipes. At all times. This could have been much worse.'

A chastened Gordon was quiet for the rest of the shift.

The more common way for patients to escape was simply to wait until they had time out of the ward, escorted or unescorted, and then just to leg it. If they did a bolter during an escorted pass, staff were warned against pursuing them, since Joe Public would not know the reason behind the pursuit and might intervene on the wrong side. I have to say that never, not once, in all my escorts, did anyone run away from me. They ran from Charlie, John, Luke – everybody else, in fact. I don't know why not me; I wasn't someone they particularly liked, and I had no special sanction against them. It was just a fact. I began to resent that no patient had fled from my clutches, as if I'd been left out of something worthwhile. Maybe they thought there was something wrong with me. It rankled, as if I'd been blackballed from the Athenaeum.

The best escapee, both in terms of the number of times he did it and of the destinations he reached, was a guy called Vic. Staff had to be extremely careful on escort with Vic. He was admitted fairly regularly because he was one of those who got better, got out and then stopped taking his meds because he assumed there was no longer anything wrong with him – the sort of patient for whom the depot injection was invented. But once he came in he tended to get better quickly. Then Charlie would take him out for a stroll and the process would begin again.

The first time out would be fine. He knew he was on trial so he kept his nose clean. But it was inevitable. We knew it and he knew it. There would come the time when he just couldn't stand it any longer; he had run out of metaphorical tissues. He would abruptly break into a sprint and hare off down the road. Occasionally he would be caught the same day, but more often he headed for the city. Sometimes he caught a train there. We had to escort him back from London on at least two occasions, the second time when he was apprehended by a bobby as he attempted to talk his way into Buck House because, as he said, he had something he needed to tell the Queen.

But his best jaunt occurred the last summer I worked in the ward. He was out walking with Clyde when he bolted. Clyde returned, informed Charlie and then informed the duty nursing officer, as per protocol. The DNO would in due course, when Vic did not return for the night, inform the police. All this was done and we waited for Vic's return. We waited six weeks. Then he was returned by the police after being refused entry to Spain. He had got himself to the city airport, dipped a passport from a passenger, gone home in the dead of night and packed a bag, then got himself on a flight to Spain. Passport checks were not so hot here, compared to Spanish immigration's. They spotted something wrong right away when Vic presented his passport. The picture was Vic's all right – he had had the sense to paste one of his own over the original. They had no problem with him being five foot six, having brown hair or green eyes. The Spaniards just didn't believe his name was Brenda.

36

And all I ask is a merry yarn from a laughing fellow-rover,
And quiet sleep and a sweet dream when the long kick's over.

John Masefield, 'Sea Fever'

Time passed – it usually does. That's what it does best, in fact. Patients were readmitted – old pals like Theo and Edward, Bernard and Stannie. Theo was most distressed to find that I was still around.

'Hey, man, you still here? Why is a cat like you still working with these fascists? You should be over the hills and far away, man, spreading love, light and peace. It's, like, totally iffy karma for you to be in here.'

And there were new admissions too. Two of my favourite people were admitted about this time – Gilbert and Popeye. Gilbert was a man in his late fifties. He had a whiff of the shabby genteel about him, a vaguely patrician air reinforced by his tweedy clothes and his insistence on being called Lord Gilbert. Schizophrenic, he was the sort of man who would have spent most of his life in an asylum in former times. Depot injections allowed him to live a quiet life in a local village, where he inhabited a house full of cats and made the occasional sortie up the street dressed like a duke's bastard. Even his speech had a tingle of the blue-blooded about it. He smoked cheroots and would sit in the Smoke Room, with his legs crossed, holding one of his old stogies like a dowager, and perfuming the place with essence of smouldering tramp. Meanwhile, he would hold forth.

'You know, it's a damned shame that a man of my calibre should be obliged to bivouac in an establishment like this. Something ought to be done about it. I've a mind to write a stiff letter to the authorities.'

'And who would they be, Gilbert?'

'*Lord* Gilbert to you, young man. And to answer your question – why, the powers that be, of course.'

Nobody, to my knowledge, ever called him Lord Gilbert seriously, but he would insist upon it. Sometimes, if things were not to his taste, he could mix the toff talk with the most foul gutter language.

'Gilbert! Teatime.'

'*Lord* Gilbert, if you please. And if you insist on addressing me simply as Gilbert, you odious little cunt, I shall kick your fucking shitpit in.'

'Okay, your lordship. Tea or coffee?'

'Tea, please. Do you have any Darjeeling?'

'Sorry, no. Sweepings of the factory floor in teabags only.'

'Well, my boy, you know what you can do with that effluent. You can stick it right up your fucking hole. Toodle pip.'

He was friendly with Popeye, whose real name was a very ordinary handle like John or Tom or something. But he was an old salt, had sailed the seven seas in his day and was wont to saunter up the ward humming, 'I'm Popeye the sailor man . . .' And he had been humming it for years. So everybody, in the ward and on the streets, called him Popeye. He was not at all offended; he answered to it quite happily. Popeye had an idiosyncratic way of talking too. His speech was peppered with quaint old naval terms.

He approached me one evening about dinnertime, having overheard that I was going upstairs to the canteen to buy my evening meal.

'Ah! You nipping up aloft, I hear? Fetch me some bacon from the galley, will you?'

I said I would. Then the trolley arrived and Popeye got a dekko at his own meal.

'Nurse!' he called to me. 'Belay my last. Adequate tuck here, thanks.'

I heard him speaking to Gordon one day.

'You know my cabin?' he was saying. 'Along the corridor here, round by the head, full sail past the desk – Treatment Room and Bathroom aids to navigation – hard ahead. Cabin Number 12. If anyone comes for me, I'll be having forty winks.'

'Anyone' was his sister, a pleasant little old lady who visited him every couple of days and brought, without fail, a copy of the *Racing Post*, a handful of betting slips, forty cigarettes and two punnets of strawberries. Betting on the horses was his hobby, and he indulged it whenever he could. He had a thing about strawberries and ate them with all the relish and selfishness of a child, handing them round to nobody. He would sit with his sister in a corner of the Dayroom, two unusually carved salt and pepper shakers, reading his racing paper, picking horses and listening absently as she fed him titbits of local gossip. Then he would write out a line and hand it to his sister. She would toddle off to put it on when she was shopping. Meanwhile, he would take his booty back to his bedroom and eat strawberries till he shat pink.

He was of an age with Gilbert and they became very friendly. Gilbert and Popeye. Might have been a duo of conceptual artists or a brace of Siamese cats. Or even an album of songs like 'Three Little Maids from School' sung by a spinach-chewing, pipe-smoking, craggy Jack Tar. Many times, for long times, times measured by a clock with no hands, they'd sit together in the Dayroom and chat.

'You know, Popeye, old chap, I've come down in the world terribly since I was a shaver. There was a time when I'd have died of mortification to think of myself in a place like this.'

'Changed days, shipmate, changed days.'

'Days always change, my friend. Always. Nothing stays the same. But there again what can you do? There's an old saw: "What cannot be cured must be endured." I suppose that's the nearest I'll ever come to a philosophy of life.'

'Life, shipmate? Life's a weary puzzle. I read that somewhere. I think. Or heard it somewhere. One of the two.'

And then they would sit silently together while the day grew old, stock-still, saying nothing, as if they were being metamorphosed slowly into two stone figures in the afternoon's grey light.

More patients were readmitted. Barry came back looking like the Last Prophet, with his hair shoulder length and his beard down to his chest. Theo was mightily impressed by this look.

'Barry looks like Lennon in the last days of the Beatles,' he said to me.

'A little,' I agreed. 'But I bet he doesn't sing like him. Barry's not too "Give Peace a Chance" really.'

'Yeah, man, but check his aura.'

'I don't believe in auras, Theo.'

'Shit, man. Everyone has their own aura, and cats that have the gift, the sight, can see the aura emanating from people. Some cats even say that it can be photographed, using a, like, ultra-sensitive and hip camera. You know, if your aura is red, it means anger or unbalanced energies, man. But white, man, white. That's the aura of perfection. Harmony. It's, like, the colour of Christ and the Buddha, you know? It clarifies every emanation. You can see the colour of your own aura in dreams, man. If you dream mainly in blue, then your aura is blue. Listen to the colour of your dreams.'

'That's from "Tomorrow Never Knows", isn't it?'

'Yeah, that's cool, man. We were talking about Lennon anyway.'

Barry didn't warm the bed too long this time either. During an interview with Dr Bankstreet he attempted to assault her. I had been in, riding shotgun with Theo, just moments before. Dr Bankstreet was trying vainly to get Theo to agree to try clozapine.

'No way, José,' he said to her. 'That shit gives you leukaemia. Hey, man, this witch is trying to give me leukaemia.'

Despite arguing a cogent case for his at least trying the drug, Dr Bankstreet knew he would have none of it. He might have been very unwell, but he was no fool. Theo was a well-read man, and he knew a thing or two about drugs. He point blank refused to consider clozapine. In the end the doc had to give up. I took Theo out.

Next up was Barry. He went in with John. They were in no longer than five minutes when the alarms started to sound. We all piled in, to find Barry with his arm round Dr Bankstreet's throat and John attempting to prise it free. About five of us tore him off the poor old doc and huckled him away for a date with his old friend, acuphase. Meanwhile, Pamela and Ursula made sure Dr Bankstreet was okay. Her neck was a little sore, but otherwise she was fine.

She smiled when we asked how she was. 'Had worse.'

Barry was transferred to a specialist unit in the city. He was moved by a well-known contract security firm. Four apes in black uniforms arrived early one morning. Barry was not yet awake. He had no idea of the treat in store for him either. The head banana of the group looked through Barry's Judas window at him.

'Is that a fork on the floor?' he asked.

'Yes, I believe it is,' I said. This guy was no slouch where cutlery was concerned.

'Why would he have a fork in his room?'

'To cut his toenails?'

The man never even cracked a smirk.

'I don't know,' I said. 'Maybe the night shift gave him one to eat a takeaway or something. Is it important?'

'I just don't want it stuck into my face when we go in,' he said. 'Wullie, you get the fork.'

One of the guards nodded.

Ah. I hadn't thought of that. Barry, as you might guess, was less than transported at the news of his removal. The four men woke him up and he was dressed, with a bag packed, in less than ten minutes. He was full of good cheer as he left us.

'Bastards, I'll get youse for this. Every last one of youse.'

And he was gone. Gone and never called me mother. Never called me anything, in fact, other than bastard. I knew it was unlikely that he would ever get any of us for it, but it was just another threat, another hassle, another major pain in the arse. And I was fed up of scraping my sores with a potsherd. I wanted more bodies on the ward. Or I wanted my own off it.

Came the Sunday and we were phoned from A & E. Geraldine took the call. They needed male staff because a patient was becoming increasingly aggressive. The man was Japanese and obviously very unwell.

'John and Luke, can you go up?' asked Geraldine.

'Aye,' said John. 'Shouldnae be a problem. If he's Japanese, he's no likely to be very big. Should be a dawdle.'

'You never heard of sumo wrestlers?' I said.

I was joking, but I was right. Yoshito was a tall man, not heavily built but solid enough to cause problems if he became violent. John and Luke were with him but in no way could they be said to be escorting him. He had come down to the Locked Ward because his wife was with him and she had persuaded him. He had run amok in A & E. Now four more male staff members arrived from other wards to provide reinforcements. This was getting to be a sickeningly familar scenario.

'He's trained in Tae Kwon Do,' whispered Luke.

'Natch,' I said. 'Nobody we get would be a third dan in origami or a kabuki actor.'

Yoshito turned out to be a very reserved and quiet man suffering from a bipolar illness. He was in the city on holiday, and had taken unwell on the way to the airport for his flight home. He was unhappy at being in the ward but his wife managed to persuade him to stay overnight to see Dr Bankstreet in the morning.

Meanwhile she booked herself into a hotel. Yoshito listened patiently while she explained all this to him in Japanese, then he nodded and went without another word into his room.

All the men sat about the Nurses' Station, on the alert.

'I think the guy's just scared,' said Clyde. 'You know, freaked at being in here.'

'Yeah, maybe. But he ripped the place apart in A & E,' said John. 'Two porters are being treated up there as a result.'

'Ach, he's quiet enough now,' said Luke.

'Yeah, but if he comes screaming out of there naked except for a white bandanna, I'm out of here,' I replied.

In fact, Yoshito remained quiet and reserved if still very obviously unhappy at being there. What got him through, I think, was the regular presence of his wife, whom he obviously trusted implicitly. He stayed a week and then Dr Bankstreet decided he should be allowed to return to Japan. Two nurses would have to go as escorts.

Now we were all used to doing escorts and transfers. Every single one of us had done dozens of them. Some were ordinary in the extreme: weapons-grade ho-hum, local runs or to the city. Others were better: two- or three-hour runs to quiet places in picturesque nooks of the Scottish countryside. One or two a year to England. I myself was involved in the London run that took Albie (of the necktie ligature) back. We were all terribly blasé and been there, done that about the whole procedure.

But this was Japan. Japan for fucksake! Jaunt of a lifetime. The ultimate transfer. Nobody was going to top this one, unless some wee green schizophrenic with an aerial in his head required escorting to the Sea of Tranquillity. We all wanted this one. Everybody. Luke was so keen he used psychological warfare to put the rest of us off.

'Yeah, it sounds great. Flight to Japan. Couple of days there. Flight back. All expenses paid. Overtime in jute sacks. But what if the big fella freaks out at 30,000 feet? Eh? What if he loses the place and starts up with the old Dolly O'Chaggie? Eh? The spin kicks or the elbow to the chops? In a plane?'

'He won't,' said Charlie. 'He's all right now. He knows he's going home. He's quite relaxed about it. Looking forward to it.'

'You want to go, Dennis?'

'Damned right I do. I should go. I'm the only one that speaks Japanese.'

'Fuck off!' sneered Luke. 'You don't speak Japanese. Having a Japanese phrasebook and calling your man Yoshito San doesn't make you a Japanese speaker.'

'Anyway, Mrs Yoshito speaks very good English.'

'Right,' said Charlie. 'Who *doesn't* want to go?'

Nobody didn't want to go. It came down to drawing lots. Charlie and Gordon went.

37

We few, we happy few, we band of brothers . . .
William Shakespeare, *Henry V*

I'd been on the ward for seven years and more. I was getting tired. I believe it's a young man's job, and staff should be on the IPCU for no more than three years at a time. Then they should be rotated to another ward, at least temporarily. Recharge their batteries. Get a different perspective. See another set of beds. Deal with another set of patients. Even if only for a year. Then maybe they could be rotated back to the Locked Ward. Certainly, it benefits from the presence of experienced staff, but everyone needs a break after a while. I certainly did. I was weary of the stress that accumulated over time, especially when there were a number of difficult patients on the ward at the same time or in quick succession.

Another aspect of the job was causing me some concern. Staffing. Now, this is not going to be a vehicle for me to get my own back against people who ground my gears over the years – and there were many of them. I don't have the patience of a saint, and I know I'm easily pissed off. I'm not going to say that I never disagreed with any of my colleagues; I did. I'm a disagreeing kind of a guy. I won't say I never fell out with people, because that's what people do, and I'm people. Nor will I claim that all of the staff I worked alongside were the finest specimens of humanity that I ever came across. Some were superb nurses, full of caring and understanding with seemingly limitless amounts of time to give to patients. Others couldn't nurse a grievance. But that's the way of the world, in all its walks. Why should nurses be any different? So. There'll be no old scores settled. One of the many things that the patients taught me was that time is too short to waste on petty vendettas. No point in replays of old matches. Use the past as a step to something better. Or different, at least.

It was staffing *complements* that concerned me. Numbers. Ratios. I have deliberately kept staff names consistent to keep people's identities secret, but in seven and a half years staff came and went regularly. My great concern was that, increasingly, they were not replaced. By the time I left the IPCU both shifts were working with about half the numbers they had had when I started. There were not enough trained nurses and not enough males. I think I've made it obvious that the ward warranted large numbers of both.

Staff were edgier, more stressed and more likely to take time off work. The domestics who had been on the ward long before my arrival said that they did not feel as safe as they had. The most important people, the patients, were not being given the level of care they should have been. Patients were arriving on the ward and staying for longer periods of time than had been the case before. There weren't enough people to speed up their care. As in many other workplaces, financial considerations were becoming too important. I'm not an idiot – I know that everybody has to work to a budget – but I am old-fashioned enough to believe that in a place like the Locked Ward patient welfare is the paramount concern. And staff welfare should follow it fairly closely.

Being the shy, retiring violet I'm not, I couldn't keep my mouth shut about this. I created a stink about it at every possible opportunity, even drafting a letter to the nursing officer in charge of psychiatric services which I let my colleagues read before mailing it to him. They all signed it. He sent a deputy to the ward, who listened to our concerns and said they would be acted upon. And – hey presto! – nothing changed.

The ward was a time bomb. One day, sure as there's shite in a goat, somebody was going to get badly hurt. I was awfully keen that it wasn't me. And then, one day when we were down to three men on the shift, an incident occurred when one of us was on lunch. Unfortunately, it wasn't me. I was one of the two left. Simon, just returned from a spell in the world, went apeshit at Pamela when she didn't provide him with a PRN the instant he demanded it. He roared abuse – we could hear him away down the ward – and made a move towards her. She set off her alarm and I went running. John came from the opposite direction. The pity is I got there first. Simon saw me coming and barged me violently into a doorway. My scholarly cranium came into contact with the frame of the door and I sat down very quickly on my beam end. I was listening to the birdies sing. John said he could see them flying in and out of my ears. He decked Simon all on his own, I later learned, and then reinforcements came running from 24. My head was not broken, but I had an egg on it for several days.

That was the one, the clincher. I thought, 'Fuck it. Who needs this?' I was a bookish and non-violent old hippy and grandfather. I wanted out of it. I'd loved it while it lasted. It was the most interesting job I'd ever had. But the time had come. My work there was done. I shouted at a few senior nurses and – abracadabra! – I was out.

38

. . . the most fatal, and dangerous exploit,
that ever I was ranged in, since first I bore arms
before the face of the enemy, as I am a gentleman and soldier.

Ben Jonson, *Every Man in his Humour*

My last shift was marked by a dramatic incident. Sometime in that last afternoon, Judy from 42 phoned down for male backup. A twenty-five-year-old male patient was going off at the deep end. He was a former soldier. (Typical. Like I say, we never had to deal with a middle-aged gay man who worked part-time on an antique stall, or a wardrobe mistress for the local repertory theatre.) In the event, it was John, Luke and Clyde who went up and fetched the bloke. It took quite a lot of guile and experience to get him downstairs. In the end they had to pretend to back away from his in-yer-face aggression and then, when he half turned away, John whisked a headlock on him and the other two helped to bear him down to the floor. Judy jagged him and he eventually calmed down long enough to do the shuffle to the lifts and then down to the bowels where we were.

When they did come in, it was all boys together. Your man was smiling wryly and joking about how a grizzled old campaigner like himself, an urban commando with years in the khaki behind him, had been outfoxed by smart ward guerillas like our boys. What a bunch of lads! A loss to the colours. Worth the watching. The stench of testosterone was choking. His name, Monty, was singularly apt. But he settled down quickly on the ward, once the usual orientation procedure had been carried out by John and Clyde. He smoked a knuckleful of fags in the courtyard and then lay down on his bunk till mess call.

It was after seven o'clock. Pamela was the senior nurse on the shift, Charlie being on holiday and Geraldine on a half-day. She was writing up her notes in the office. Gordon and I were in there too, helping her by talking about the weekend football results. She looked up from her writing, turned and checked the wall clock. She asked if anyone was doing the teas. We said Ursula and Rona were.

'Lock the courtyard, somebody; it's getting dark.'

Gordon stood to do it. We heard the courtyard door grate open, and then Gordon's voice call to someone still out there. There was a brief dialogue and then Gordon came back into the office.

'Monty's out there. Refusing to come in. Says he's got a knife and he'll use it on anyone who tries to manhandle him indoors.'

'Oh God,' said Pamela and stood up. 'Dennis, get the boys.'

She went to the courtyard door and stuck her head out. I looked out the window. Monty was in the far corner of the courtyard, having a skulk and a sulk combined, arms crossed like Napoleon in the wilderness.

'Monty?'

'Stay away. I'll stick the first bastard that comes near me,' he shouted back. I went for the boys.

John, Luke and Clyde returned to the courtyard door with me.

'You try and talk some sense to him, John,' said Pamela. 'He seemed to get on with you earlier.'

'Where is he?' asked John. There was a fair well of darkness out there in the yard by that time.

'In the far corner. By Simon's window.'

John cautiously turtled his head out of the door and looked around. Then he stepped out into the yard, staying hard by the open door.

'Monty! It's me, John.'

'You better not come anywhere near me again, you bastard. I'm carrying and I'll use it.'

'You need to come into the ward, Monty,' said John. 'It's getting dark. The tea's on the go.'

'Fuck you and the tea!'

'There's five of us,' called John. 'If we need to come out mob-handed to get you, we will. We'd rather you just came in by yourself. But if you insist, we'll come out and get you.'

'I don't care if there's a *hundred* and five of you. The first one near me will get fucking plunged.'

To reinforce Monty's threat, a small pebble, obviously from one of the planters in the yard, whistled by John's head and smacked off the glass of the courtyard door.

'Come in, John,' said Pamela. When he did, she locked the door. 'The police can deal with this if he's armed.'

'Think he *is* armed?' asked Luke.

'He's got something in his hand, for sure,' said John. 'He was waving it about at me as we spoke.'

'A knife?' asked Pamela.

'Could be,' agreed John.

Pamela went into the office and called the police, explaining that one of the patients in the Locked Ward, an ex-soldier, was in the yard, refusing to re-enter the ward as instructed and threatening staff with a knife. She was told there would be police backup there as soon as possible.

Fair play to them!

Two officers from (I assume) an armed response unit came in and recced the site and then, before you could say CO19, the place was hoaching with officers in helmets, body armour, stab vests and fire-resistant overalls, with torches, batons, pepper spray and, I'm sure, tear gas. But the thing was, these guys just kept coming. Two, three, four, five sprinting along the ward corridor to occupy the bedrooms giving on to the yard. Six, seven, eight following Clyde round to the long service corridor behind the courtyard, where there was an emergency door, always kept locked. Nine, ten standing at the ward door to the yard. *Tramp tramp tramp* in the corridor outside the ward, then *tramp tramp tramp* as they sprinted away to occupy positions in the windows of the corridors above the yard. It was like the final scenes of *Butch Cassidy*. Then four men went out into the courtyard to bring him in. I watched from the office. The walls of the hospital were blocks of lit windows. There were three faces in every window.

They brought Monty in without too much trouble. He was carrying a Swiss army knife. He might have tweezered John to death, I suppose, or sharpened a pencil for him. Or even opened a bottle of Aloxe-Corton to toast their new friendship. Unlikely to have done him any lasting damage, though.

Still, it was an interesting way to leave the ward. Nice to go out on a cinematic high.

39

One who never turned his back but marched breast forward,
Never doubted clouds would break,
Never dreamed, though right were worsted, wrong would triumph,
Held we fall to rise, are baffled to fight better,
Sleep to wake.

Robert Browning, 'Epilogue to Asolando'

A final word about the patients . . .

I learned as much from the patients I met in just over seven years as I have in the rest of a (so far) reasonably long life – from teachers, university lecturers, pundits or gurus of any kind. I hope I helped some of the patients a little. I know they furthered my education in many things.

The greatest lesson I learned from them was the indomitability of the human spirit. I'd read much about it in fiction and seen it filleted in the movies. But I saw the real thing, and lived beside it, week by week and month by month, in the ward. No fictional narratives, no cinematic happy endings, just life *as it is* for some. Despite suffering from the most hair-raising, sometimes completely incapacitating illnesses, people's determination to rise above the abyss was utterly remarkable. People with the most appalling conditions faced their horrors and still made a life for themselves. If they could not be granted a silver-bullet miraculous cure, they settled for a grain-by-grain improvement, no matter how long it took, and no matter how regular the setbacks.

As Samuel Beckett says in 'Worstward Ho': 'Ever tried. Ever failed. No matter. Try Again. Fail again. Fail better.' Whether they were trying to get access to their children, deal with tenancy difficulties, get over a bereavement, keep a relationship going or just find money from somewhere when it seemed they had none, their bravery and resourcefulness were simply staggering.

Time and again, some patients were readmitted to the ward. Time and again, they faced their trials with courage and hope. Time and again, their hopes were dashed. And they turned round and set their faces to the wind yet again.

What's not to admire?

This book is primarily a tribute to all of them. And so it is to the patients that I dedicate it – those extraordinary, sometimes infuriating, often exhilarating, individuals without whom . . .